PHARMACEUTICAL
CALCULATIONS

PHARMACEUTICAL CALCULATIONS
Third Edition

JOEL L. ZATZ
Department of Pharmaceutics
College of Pharmacy
Rutgers University
Piscataway, New Jersey

A Wiley-Interscience Publication
JOHN WILEY & SONS, INC.
New York   Chichester   Brisbane   Toronto   Singapore

This text is printed on acid-free paper.

Library of Congress Cataloging in Publication Data:
Zatz, Joel L., 1935–
    Pharmaceutical calculations / Joel Zatz. — 3rd ed.
       p.   cm.
    Includes index.
    ISBN 0-471-10623-2
    1. Pharmaceutical arithmetic. I. Title.
    RS57.Z37 1994
    615'.1'01513—dc20   94-23061

Printed in the United States of America

10 9 8 7 6 5 4 3 2 1

To Arline and David

With love, thanks and a vision of tomorrow.

CONTENTS

PREFACE

Preparation of a new edition of *Pharmaceutical Calculations* was mandated by the evolution in pharmacy practice that has taken place during the past decade. My goal was to respond to these changes by updating the topics that serve as the traditional core of the subject, eliminating antiquated examples, and adding new chapters on subject areas of practical importance. At the same time, I wanted to retain the approach and essential features of previous editions, which have been used successfully by pharmacy students for over 20 years. In line with this, a number of changes have been made in this edition. Certain units and abbreviations have been updated. Learning objectives have been included at the beginning of each chapter. New chapters deal with osmolarity, isoosmotic solutions, parenteral nutrition, radioactive decay and drug stability. Several topics not requiring separate chapters have been included in an Appendix. Most problems utilizing the apothecary system, which has all but disappeared from practical use, have been removed from the text.

Dimensional analysis and direct approaches in problem solving are emphasized. Accuracy requirements, which depend on the particular application, are indicated and estimation as a means of preventing gross errors is encouraged. Alligation is no longer included as a calculation method. This mathematical crutch was useful at a time when many students did not know algebra, but has no justification today.

As with previous editions, this text can stand alone in the self-instructional mode or serve as a primary or supplementary text in a formal course. The programmed format permits self-paced learning. Answers to all problems are given, providing students with immediate feedback regarding their progress. A set of review questions at the end of each chapter allows students to see how well they have mastered the subject matter.

I want to thank Dr. Bert Wagner for reviewing the chapter on parenteral nutrition and all of the students and colleagues who commented on the book and made suggestions for revision. The assistance of my editor, Betty Sun, the production editor, Bob Hilbert, and the rest of the Wiley staff is also appreciated.

TO THE STUDENT

This is probably not your first encounter with a programmed text. In that case, you will recognize that each chapter contains a series of sections, called frames, in which the elements of a topic unfold step by step. Along the way, you have to answer questions that check your understanding. The answer is always available, so you can quickly tell whether you're on the right track or not.

One principle involved in this approach to teaching is active learning. This means that the work you do in attacking problems and thinking about your answers helps you to understand and remember, making it easier for you the next time you come across another problem in which the same logic and ideas are important. To just read the problems and answers or glance ahead at the solutions to the problems defeats the process.

Most every frame contains a dashed line. Take an index card and place it on the frame you're working on so that it covers everything below the dashed line. (That's where the answer is.) Read the information in the frame and work on the question or questions in the space provided. When you're done, check your answer. If you are correct, move on to the next frame. If not, try the problem again before consulting the solution. You may uncover your error and be able to do it right the second time. If you still can't get it, you may want to go back a few frames to see if there is something you missed. If all else fails, look at the solution. You may also want to consult the solution if you struggled to get the right answer and wondered if a more direct approach is available.

I am assuming that you can perform the usual arithmetic operations of addition, subtraction, multiplication and division and that you can solve simple algebraic and exponential equations.

Outlines of certain techniques are provided in case you have gotten rusty and need to review. Working through the problems that are provided will usually get you back on track.

Some questions will be easy for you and you'll zoom through the text. Difficult spots will take more time; in any case, stick with it and take as much time as you need to work through the material until you understand it and can handle the problems. Happy problem solving!

PHARMACEUTICAL CALCULATIONS

CHAPTER ONE

SOME BASICS

In their daily practice, pharmacists are called upon repeatedly to make certain kinds of calculations. They must determine the quantities of materials required to fill prescriptions and make up formulas. The dosage of each medicament that is dispensed must be checked, since the pharmacist is legally accountable for an overdose. The fact that most pharmaceutical manufacturing is performed outside the pharmacy does not in any way lessen the pharmacist's responsibility.

Modern drugs are effective, potent, and therefore potentially toxic. Knowing "how to" calculate the amount of each drug and "how to" combine them is not sufficient. Put yourself in the place of a newly created widow whose husband was the victim of an overdose caused by a careless error in calculation. It would not comfort you to have the pharmacist say, "Don't be sad. I knew how to do that calculation. I used the right method."

Of course, dispensing an underdose is not satisfactory either. The drug(s) given will probably not elicit the desired therapeutic effect and will therefore be of no benefit to the patient. Clearly, the only satisfactory approach is one that is completely free of error. Absolute accuracy is our goal.

Since our goal when performing calculations is the correct answer, it is logical to suppose that any rational approach to a problem that results in the correct answer is acceptable. While this is true, some approaches are more rational than others. Try to use a method that requires as few steps as possible. The simplest, most direct pathway to the solution allows less opportunity for error in computation than does one that is roundabout.

In the first half of this chapter, we will go into some manipulative techniques basic to your calculations. I am going to assume that you can add, subtract, multiply, and divide; that you can work with decimals and fractions; and that you can solve simple algebraic expressions. You will probably find that you are already familiar with all or most of the techniques covered. When that is so, you will make rapid progress through the program. But if you need further review or instruction, they will be provided.

We will see how units participate in arithmetic operations and how we can take advantage of this property in our calculations. We will review proportion, estimation, rounding, and power-of-10 notation.

The second half of the chapter deals with measurement and its accuracy. We will discuss the tolerances permitted and notations used in describing measured values obtained by the pharmacist.

Learning objectives: after completing this chapter the student should be able to

1. Perform mathematical operations on units.
2. Use statements of equivalence to convert measurements from one unit to another.
3. Use proportion as a calculation tool.
4. Estimate results using rounding and power-of-10 notation.
5. Express tolerances in terms of amounts and percentages.
6. State the accepted tolerances for prescription and manufacturing calculations.
7. Calculate minimum weighable and measurable quantities for various instruments used by the pharmacist.

---

1. In compounding prescriptions, the pharmacist deals with measured quantities. The magnitude of each such quantity is expressed as the product of a number and a unit. The unit name specifies the scale of measurement. My pencil, for example, is 5 inches (in.) long. I may also say that it is 12.7 centimeters (cm) long. Changing the scale of measurement (unit) causes the multiplying number to change as well. Thus, in describing any measured quantity, it is necessary to specify the unit used. The unit is an integral part of the designation of a value that is either measured directly or calculated from measured data. It must not be permitted to drop off or fade away during calculation.

   It is sometimes found that the units in which a measured quantity is expressed are not convenient for the user. For example, an American traveling in Mexico learns that the distance from Mexico City to Cuernavaca is 88 kilometers (km). Before undertaking the trip, the traveler may wish to convert this distance into the equivalent number of miles (mi), a unit with which she is more familiar. To perform the conversion, it is necessary to know that

1 mi = 1.6 km

This mathematical statement relates the two units to each other; it is a statement of equivalence.

In the spaces provided, write a statement of equivalence for the following:

A.   inches and feet (ft)
B.   grams (g) and milligrams (mg)
C.   dollars and cents

_____

A.   1 ft = 12 in. (or 1 in. = 1/12 ft)
B.   1 g = 1000 mg (or 1 mg = 0.001 g)
C. $1 = 100¢ (or 1¢ = $0.01)

---

2.   Units may be multiplied and divided in much the same way as numbers or algebraic symbols. For example, a unit of force is the newton (N). Since

force = mass × acceleration

$$N = kg \times m/s^2$$

so that

$$N = \frac{(kg)\,(m)}{s^2}$$

If the same unit appears in both the numerator and denominator, they will cancel each other. For example, the newton/meter may be taken as a unit of surface force:

$$N = \frac{(kg)\,(m)}{s^2}$$

$$\frac{N}{m} = \frac{(kg)\,(m)}{(s^2)\,(m)} = \frac{kg}{s^2}$$

Perform the operations indicated. Cancel units where appropriate.

A.   cm × g =

B. $mm \times \dfrac{1}{mm} =$

C.   lb × oz/lb =

————————————————————————

A.   (cm) (g) or (g) (cm)

B. $\dfrac{mm}{mm}$ = 1

C.   lb × oz/lb = oz

———

3.   We have not yet solved the problem of our American tourist who wishes to know how many miles are represented by 88 km. To find out, we make use of our statement of equivalence in this way:

$$88 \ km \ \times \frac{1 \ mi}{1.6 \ km} = 55 \ mi$$

Let us stop and examine the fraction $\dfrac{1 \ mi}{1.6 \ km}$. Since the numerator is equal to the denominator, the value of this fraction is unity, or 1. Multiplication by unity will not change the distance represented by 88 km, only the way in which this distance is expressed, which is exactly our intention.

Identify, with a check, which of the following fractions have a value of unity.

A.   10 mm/1 cm
B.   1 qt/2 pt
C.   1 lb/8 oz
D.   1 in./12 ft
E.   2 yd/6 ft

————————————————————————

A, B, and E have a value of unity.

Solutions:

A.   1 cm = 10 mm. Since the numerator and denominator are equivalent, the value of the fraction is unity.
B.   1 qt = 2 pt. The numerator and denominator are equivalent.
C.   There are 16 oz, not 8 oz, in a pound. The numerator is not equivalent to the denominator, and the fraction does not have a value of unity.
D.   If you missed this, look again: 1 ft = 12 in. but 1 in. does not equal 12 ft. The numerator and denominator are not equivalent.

E.   Since 1 yd = 3 ft, 2 yd = 6 ft. The numerator and
denominator of the fraction are equivalent.

4.   A weight-watcher wishes to know how many grams are
equivalent to 4 oz of beef. State which of the following operations
will lead to the correct answer and why the others are not correct
(1 oz = 28.4 g).

A. $4 \text{ oz} \times \dfrac{1 \text{ oz}}{28.4 \text{ g}} =$

B. $1 \text{ oz} \times \dfrac{28.4 \text{ g}}{1 \text{ oz}} =$

C. $4 \text{ oz} \times \dfrac{14.2 \text{ g}}{1 \text{ oz}} =$

D. $4 \text{ oz} \times \dfrac{28.4 \text{ g}}{1 \text{ oz}} =$

D is correct because the ounces will cancel and 4 oz will be
converted to grams. In A, the multiplying fraction is inverted,
leading to incorrect units (oz^2/g) in the result. In B, the quantity
to be converted is not the desired quantity; from this expression,
we will find the number of grams in 1 oz, not 4 oz, of beef. In C,
the value of the multiplying fraction is not equal to unity. This
will alter the value of the weight of the meat, resulting in an
incorrect answer.

5.   To summarize, conversion of a quantity from one unit system to
another is accomplished by multiplication of that quantity by a
fraction whose value is unity. The denominator of the fraction is
given in terms of the original units, while the numerator is
expressed in terms of the desired units.
    How many fluid ounces are there in 4/5 qt of Scotch whiskey?
(Recall that 1 qt contains 32 fluidounces.)

25.6 fluidounces

Solution:

$$0.8 \text{ qt} \times \frac{32 \text{ fluidounces}}{1 \text{ qt}} = 25.6 \text{ fluidounces}$$

6. Sometimes, the equivalence between the units given and the units desired is not known. Say, for example, that we wish to convert 17 ft to meters. Although we do not know the number of feet in 1 m, we do know that 1 m = 39.4 in. and 1 ft = 12 in. We may therefore first convert feet to inches and then inches to meters. But rather than treat our problem as two separate parts, we may set it up as follows:

$$17 \text{ ft} \times \frac{12 \text{ in.}}{1 \text{ ft}} \times \frac{1 \text{ m}}{39.4 \text{ in.}} = 5.18 \text{ m}$$

The first fraction converts feet to inches; the second converts inches to meters. Notice that all units except for meters cancel out. There is no change in the value of the length represented by "17 ft." This technique may be extended to any number of successive conversions.

7. How many fluidounces are there in 1.75 liters (L)? (1 L = 1000 mL; 1 fluidounce = 29.6 mL)

--- --- --- --- --- --- --- --- --- --- ---

59.1 fluidounces

Solution:

$$1.75 \text{ L} \times 1000 \text{ mL/L} \times \frac{1 \text{ fluidounce}}{29.6 \text{ mL}} = 59.1 \text{ fluidounces}$$

8. If a mercury barometer reads 30.3 in., what is the pressure in atmospheres (atm)? (1 in. = 2.54 cm; 1 atm = 76 cm)

- - - - - - - - - - - - - - - - - -

1.01 atm

Solution:

$$30.3 \text{ in.} \times \frac{2.54 \text{ cm}}{1 \text{ in.}} \times \frac{1 \text{ atm}}{76 \text{ cm}} = 1.01 \text{ atm}$$

9.   Here are some more practice problems.

A.   One gallon equals 231 in.^{3}. If there are 1728 in.^{3} in a cubic foot, how many gallons are there in 3.5 ft^3?

B.   If there are 220 yd to a furlong and 1 furlong = 10 chains, how many yards are there in 3.7 chains?

C.   There are 2.20 lb in a kilogram. If a man weighs 180 lb, how many kilograms is that?

- - - - - - - - - - - - - - - - - -

A.   26.2 gal
B.   81.4 yd
C.   81.8 kg

10. Another technique useful in solving arithmetical problems is that of proportion. You are probably familiar with this method, and the problems that follow should present no difficulty to you. A

brief review is provided in case you have gotten rusty. Remember to write all units and to make certain that the expressions on opposite sides of the equals sign have the same units.

    Do all of the problems, using proportion, before verifying your answers.

A. $\dfrac{1\ kg}{\$3.50} = \dfrac{j}{\$2.00}$ $j =$ _____ kg

B. If 127 paper clips weigh 1.5 oz, how many paper clips will weigh 1/2 lb?

C. An analytical instrument that is in constant use needs a new battery every 73 days. How many batteries will be required for a year?

— — — — — — — — — — — — — — — — — —

  A. 0.571 kg
  B. 677 paper clips
  C. 5 batteries

(If you breezed through these problems, proceed directly to frame 16. For a review of proportion, go on to frame 11.)

11. Proportions are useful in those situations where two properties are directly related to each other. For example, if a drug costs 5¢ per gram, 2 g will cost 10¢. The two properties, cost and amount of drug, are directly related to each other. If the quantity of drug is increased five times, the cost will increase five times. If the amount of drug is cut in half, the cost will be halved also. If we wanted to know the cost of 12.5 g of this drug, we could write

$$\frac{1 \text{ g}}{5 \cancel{c}} = \frac{12.5 \text{ g}}{j}$$

This equation states, "If 1 g of a drug costs 5¢, then 12.5 g will cost j." Notice that the same units are found on both sides of the equality. The ratio on the left describes the known relationship between the related properties. The ratio on the right describes the unknown situation. The two ratios are equal to each other because there is a fixed relationship between cost and weight.

One sodium bicarbonate tablet contains 300 mg of the drug; we wish to find the number of tablets that will contain 1500 mg of sodium bicarbonate. Which of the following proportions will lead to the correct solution? Why are the others not correct?

A. $\dfrac{1 \text{ tablet}}{300 \text{ mg}} = \dfrac{1500 \text{ mg}}{j}$

B. $\dfrac{1 \text{ tablet}}{1500 \text{ mg}} = \dfrac{j}{300 \text{ mg}}$

C. $\dfrac{1 \text{ tablet}}{300 \text{ mg}} = \dfrac{j}{1500 \text{ mg}}$

C is correct. The ratio on the left describes the known information; that on the right, the unknown situation. Both ratios have the same units. A is incorrect because the same units do not appear in both sides of the equality (tablets/mg do not equal mg/tablet). B is incorrect because the first ratio states that 1500 mg are found in each tablet (1500 mg and 300 mg are reversed). Although the units appear to be correct, the numbers have been jumbled.

---

12. To solve a proportion,

$$\frac{a}{b} = \frac{c}{d}$$

we make use of the fact that the product of the first and last terms (a and d) is equal to that of the two central terms (b and c). That is, $a \times d = c \times b$. To return to our problem,

$$\frac{1 \text{ tablet}}{300 \text{ mg}} = \frac{j}{1500 \text{ mg}}$$

$$(1 \text{ tablet}) (1500 \text{ mg}) = j(300 \text{ mg})$$

$$j = \frac{(1 \text{ tablet}) (1500 \text{ mg})}{300 \text{ mg}} = 5 \text{ tablets}$$

A formula for 42 capsules (caps) calls for 300 mg of a drug. Using proportion, find how many milligrams of the drug would be needed to make 24 capsules.

_ _

171 mg

Solution:

$$\frac{300 \text{ mg}}{42 \text{ caps}} = \frac{j}{24 \text{ caps}}$$

$$j = \frac{300 \text{ mg} \times 24 \text{ caps}}{42 \text{ caps}} = 171 \text{ mg}$$

---

13. If 12.0 g of a powder occupy 7.00 mL, how many milliliters will be taken up by 150 g?

_ _

87.5 mL

Solution:

$$\frac{12.0 \text{ g}}{7.00 \text{ mL}} = \frac{150 \text{ g}}{j}$$

$$j = \frac{7 \text{ mL} \times 150 \text{ g}}{12 \text{ g}} = 87.5 \text{ mL}$$

---

14. If a chemical costs $14 per kilogram, how many kilograms could be purchased for $128?

— —

9.14 kg

Solution:

$$\frac{1 \text{ kg}}{\$14} = \frac{j}{\$128}$$

$$j = \frac{1 \text{ kg} \times \$128}{\$14} = 9.14 \text{ kg}$$

---

15. If you want more practice, try these problems.

A. A set of AA batteries lasts 3 hours (h) and 30 minutes in a radio under constant use. How many hours will the radio play on 14 sets of batteries?

B. If 4 chairs in an auditorium occupy 17 ft^2, how many square feet are needed to accommodate 304 chairs?

C. Five hundred penicillin tablets cost $43.09. What is the cost of 48 tablets?

— —

A.   49 h
B.   1292 ft^2
C. $4.14

16. Because of the importance of accuracy in performing
calculations, it's a good idea to check all results. You might think
that this is unnecessary, since calculators are in such widespread
use. One problem with calculating machines is that we tend to
take their results for granted, without thinking about them. An
error in entering data is liable to go unnoticed just because we
have so much confidence in the infallibility of these machines. For
safety's sake, it is necessary to check every calculation in some
way, to make sure that the result is reasonable.
    One kind of check is particularly useful in preventing errors
of large magnitude such as misplacement of the decimal point.
The method to which I am referring is that of estimation, using
rounded values. The first step in this process is to round all values
to one figure. The figure is kept as it appears in the original
number if the figure following it is 4 or less. The single figure is
promoted to the next higher number if it is followed by a 5 or
higher number. For example,

4.27 rounded to one figure is 4
0.37 rounded to one figure is 0.4
3508 rounded to one figure is 4000
0.00949 rounded to one figure is 0.009

Round to one figure.

A.   72
B.   0.08294
C.   0.452
D.   0.75
E.   820

———————————————————————

A.   70
B.   0.08
C.   0.5
D.   0.8
E.   800

17. Before attempting to obtain the exact solution to a problem,
estimate the answer. After solving the problem, compare the
exact solution with the estimate. Unless they are reasonably close
to each other, both should be recalculated. Unfortunately, it is

necessary to know how to do the problem in order to come up with an estimate. It is therefore possible to "solve" a problem incorrectly and to have that wrong answer check against the estimate. Estimation is helpful in preventing errors but is not infallible. The estimated answer is found by rounding off the quantities involved in the calculation to one figure and then computing the result.

A formula for 42 capsules calls for 180 mg of sucrose. To estimate the amount of sucrose per capsule, round 42 capsules to 40 capsules and 180 mg to 200 mg:

200 mg/40 caps = 5 mg/caps

(The exact answer is 4.28 mg per capsule.)

---

18. A certain tablet contains 32.5 mg of phenobarbital. Estimate the number of milligrams of phenobarbital in 24 tablets.

_____

600 mg

Solution:

30 mg/tablet × 20 tablets = 600 mg

The exact answer is 780 mg. You may think that 600 mg is rather a poor estimate, but it is good enough to tell you that your answer is in the ballpark. Certainly, if you were to solve the problem and come up with an answer of 78 mg or 7800 mg, you would realize that an error had been made.

---

19. A liquid costs $3.27 per pint. Estimate the cost of 418 pints.

_____

$1200.

Solution:

$3/pt × 400 pt = $1200. (The exact answer is $1366.86.)

---

20. It is often convenient to use power-of-10 notation in calculation. You should already be familiar with this way of writing numbers. In "standard notation" a number is expressed as the product of a multiplier between 1 and 10 inclusive, and a power of 10. The number in example B, below, is in standard notation. As a review, try the following examples.

A. $10^2 =$
B. $5.7 \times 10^{-3} =$
C. $60 \times 10^6 =$
D. $3 \times 10^1 =$
E. $70,000 = 7 \times 10^?$
F. $0.02 = 2 \times$
G. $20 = 2 \times$
H. $10^3 \times 10^2 =$
I. $10^3/10^1 =$
J. $\dfrac{10^0 \times 10^4}{10^3} =$
K. $10^1 \times 10^{-3} =$
L. $(3 \times 10^2) \times (2 \times 10^3) =$
M. $\dfrac{(16 \times 10^2) \times (2 \times 10^{-4})}{(4 \times 10^{-1}) \times 10^1} =$
N. $(3.83 \times 10^{3)} - (2.6 \times 10^{2)} =$

_____

A. 100
B. 0.0057
C. 60,000,000
D. 30
E. 4
F. 10^{-2}
G. 10^1
H. 10^5
I. 10^2
J. 10^1
K. 10^{-2}
L. 6×10^5
M. 8×10^{-2}
N. 3.57×10^3

(If you completed these successfully, go on to frame 27. If you had difficulty or feel a bit unsure of yourself, go to frame 21 for a review of power-of-10 notation.)

21. To change 10 raised to a power, n, to a natural number, first write the figure "1" and then, if the exponent (power) is $+n$, move the decimal point to the right n places, but if the exponent is $-n$, move the decimal point n places to the left.

$$10^4 (n = +4) = 10,000$$
$$10^{-3} (n = -3) = 0.001$$
$$10^0 (n = 0) = 1$$

Complete the following:

A. $10^2 =$
B. $10^{-2} =$
C. $10^1 =$
D. $10^6 =$
E. $10^{-4} =$
F. $10^{-6} =$
G. $10^0 =$
H. $10^{-1} =$

_____

A. 100
B. 0.01
C. 10
D. 1,000,000
E. 0.0001
F. 0.000001
G. 1
H. 0.1

22. To change the product of a power of 10 and a multiplying number to a single natural number, first write the multiplying number and then, if the exponent is $+n$, move the decimal point to the right n places; but if the exponent is $-n$, move the decimal point n places to the left.

$$4.2 \times 10^2 (n = +2) = 420$$
$$37.5 \times 10^{-3} (n = -3) = 0.0375$$
$$0.29 \times 10^1 (n = +1) = 2.9$$

Change the following expressions to a single natural number:

A. $5 \times 10^1 =$

B. $1.47 \times 10^4 =$
C. $1.2 \times 10^{-3} =$
D. $14 \times 10^{-2} =$
E. $5.7 \times 10^6 =$
F. $0.002 \times 10^3 =$

— — — — — — — — — — — — — — — — — — —

A.   50
B.   14,700
C.   0.0012
D.   0.14
E.   5,700,000
F.   2

---

23. To change a natural number to the product of a power of 10 and a multiplier, write the number and move the decimal point as many places as desired. If the decimal point is moved to the left, the exponent is a positive number equal to the number of places the decimal point is moved. If the decimal point is moved to the right, the exponent is a negative number equal to the number of places the decimal point is moved. Thus:

   1. $300 = 300 \times 10^0 = 3 \times 10^2$
   2. $50,000 = 50,000 \times 10^0 = 5 \times 10^4$
   3. $0.087 = 0.087 \times 10^0 = 87 \times 10^{-3}$
   4. $127 = 127 \times 10^0 = 1.27 \times 10^2$
   5. $0.35 = 0.35 \times 10^0 = 3.5 \times 10^{-1}$

   Notice that all of the examples have been written in standard notation (in which the decimal point follows the first number in the multiplier) except for example 3.
   Fill in the proper exponent in the following expressions:

A. $480 = 4.8 \times 10$
B. $0.0095 = 9.5 \times 10$
C. $38 = 3.8 \times 10$
D. $0.013 = 1.3 \times 10$
E. $1000 = 1 \times 10$
F. $0.000001 = 1 \times 10$
G. $0.728 = 72.8 \times 10$
H. $27 = 0.27 \times 10$

— — — — — — — — — — — — — — — — — — —

A.   2
B.   −3

C. 1
D. −2
E. 3
F. −6
G. −2
H. 2

---

24. When multiplying powers of 10, add exponents. When dividing, subtract exponents.

$$10^2 \times 10^4 = 10^6$$

$$10^{-3} \times 10^2 = 10^{-1}$$

$$10^4/10^3 = 10^1$$

$$10^1/10^4 = 10^{-3}$$

$$\frac{10^1 \times 10^5}{10^2} = \frac{10^6}{10^2} = 10^4$$

Try these:

A. $10^6 \times 10^1 =$
B. $10^6 \times 10^{-3} =$
C. $\dfrac{10^2}{10^3} =$
D. $\dfrac{10^4}{10^1 \times 10^3} =$
E. $\dfrac{10^2 \times 10^{-1} \times 10^3}{10^3 \times 10^{-4}} =$

— — — — — — — — — — — — — — — — — —

A. 10^7
B. 10^3
C. 10^{-1}
D. $10^0 = 1$
E. 10^5

---

25. When multiplying expressions containing powers of 10, add exponents and multiply the other numbers as usual. When performing division, subtract exponents and divide the other numbers as usual.

$$(3 \times 10^1) \times (2 \times 10^2) = (3 \times 2) \times (10^1 \times 10^2) = 6 \times 10^3$$

$$\frac{9 \times 10^2}{3 \times 10^4} = 3 \times 10^{-2}$$

$$\frac{(4 \times 10^1) \times (3 \times 10^{-2})}{(2 \times 10^{-2}) \times (1 \times 10^4)} = \frac{(4 \times 3) \times (10^1 \times 10^{-2})}{(2 \times 1) \times (10^{-2} \times 10^4)}$$

$$= \frac{12 \times 10^{-1}}{2 \times 10^2} = 6 \times 10^{-3} = 0.006$$

Complete the following, expressing the answer in powers of 10:

A. $\dfrac{(3 \times 10^2) \times (4 \times 10^1)}{2 \times 10^{-1}} =$

B. $\dfrac{70,000 \times 0.8 \times 30}{20 \times 600 \times 0.02} =$

- -

A. 6×10^4
B. 7×10^3

26. When expressions containing powers of 10 are to be added or subtracted, all expressions must contain the same power of 10.

$$(3.4 \times 10^2) + (5.2 \times 10^2) = 8.6 \times 10^2$$

$$(2.5 \times 10^2) + (8 \times 10^1) = ?$$

The latter operation cannot be performed unless one of the exponents is changed so that both are the same. We may change both to 10^1:

$$2.5 \times 10^2 = ? \times 10^1$$

Since the exponent will be reduced by 1, the decimal point must be moved one place to the right. (The exponential portion of the term is divided by 10; the multiplier must be multiplied by 10 to keep the value of the number from changing.) Thus

$$2.5 \times 10^2 = 25 \times 10^1$$

Now we can add:

$$(25 \times 10^1) + (8 \times 10^1) = 33 \times 10^1 = 330$$

or both may be changed to contain 10^2:

$$8 \times 10^1 = ? \times 10^2$$

The exponent will be increased by 1, so the decimal point will move one place to the left:

$$8 \times 10^1 = 0.8 \times 10^2$$

$$(2.5 \times 10^2) + (0.8 \times 10^2) = 3.3 \times 10^2 = 330$$

Complete the following:

A. $(3.7 \times 10^1) - (2.5 \times 10^1) =$
B. $(12.4 \times 10^2) + (4.20 \times 10^3) =$
C. $(6.0 \times 10^{-1}) - (5 \times 10^{-2}) =$

_____

A. 1.2×10^1
B. $5.44 \times 10^3 = 54.4 \times 10^2 = 5440$
C. 0.55

---

27. Power-of-10 notation makes it easy to keep track of the decimal point in a complex calculation. It also comes in handy when estimating. Consider this example:

$$\frac{387 \times 14}{82.2} = ?$$

To estimate the answer, round to one figure and write using power-of-10 notation:

387 is rounded to 4×10^2

14 is rounded to 1×10^1

82.2 is rounded to 8×10^1

Thus

$$\frac{(4 \times 10^2) \times (1 \times 10^1)}{8 \times 10^1} = \frac{4 \times 10^3}{8 \times 10^1} = 0.5 \times 10^2 = 50$$

Estimate the answer to these problems, using power-of-10 notation:

A. $\dfrac{2700 \times 0.008}{0.563} =$

B. $\dfrac{5070}{1,000,000 \times 0.0132} =$

- -

A. $\dfrac{(3 \times 10^3) \times (8 \times 10^{-3})}{6 \times 10^{-1}} = 40$

B. $\dfrac{5 \times 10^3}{(1 \times 10^6) \times (1 \times 10^{-2})} = 0.5$

---

28. In all of the problems that you will encounter from now on, estimate the result. Arrive at your estimate mentally, if possible. Use power-of-10 notation, when you need it, to keep track of the decimal point. Write down the estimate. Then perform the calculation using the estimate as a check. Use this procedure in doing the following problems:

A. A formula for vitamin B_{12} tablets calls for 0.020 mg of the vitamin per tablet. How many milligrams are required to make 350,000 tablets?

B. A pharmacist bought a 500-g bottle of a drug for $3.79. What is the cost of 33 g of that drug?

C. A chemical costs 3.3¢ per milligram. What is the cost of 8.8 g? (1 g = 1000 mg)

- -

A.   7000 mg
B.   25¢
C $290.40

Solutions:

A.   0.020 mg/tablet × 350,000 tablets = 7000 mg

[Estimate: $(2 \times 10^{-2}) \times (4 \times 10^{5}) = 8 \times 10^{3} = 8000$ mg]

B. $\dfrac{500 \text{ g}}{\$3.79} = \dfrac{33 \text{ g}}{j}$

$j = \$0.25 = 25$¢

$\left(\text{Estimate:} j = \dfrac{3 \times 10^{1} \times 4}{5 \times 10^{2}} = 2.4 \times 10^{-1} = \$0.24 \right)$

C.   8.8 g × 1000 mg/g = 8800 mg

$\dfrac{3.3 ¢}{1 \text{ mg}} = \dfrac{j}{8800 \text{ mg}}$

$j = \$290.40$

[Estimate: $j = 3 \times 9 \times 10^{3} = 27,000$¢ (i.e., $= \$270$)]

29. We began by emphasizing the necessity for accuracy in calculation, and we explored some techniques to minimize calculation error. It is important to realize, though, that coupled to nearly every calculation is a physical measurement. Solid drug materials are usually handled in powdered form and are weighed on a balance. Liquids and solutions may also be weighed, but most often they are measured by volume in a device such as a graduate or pipet. All instruments have limitations. Some balances are intended to be more sensitive than others. Different volumetric instruments may not achieve the same level of

accuracy. The particular instrument and technique chosen for a measurement depend on the degree of accuracy that is required.

---

30. All measurements are subject to error. When an instrument is faulty or when a reagent is incorrectly prepared, systematic errors (always positive or always negative) will be introduced and the results will be "biased." Errors of this type may be minimized by checking equipment for proper function, by using care in handling materials and running suitable checks where possible, and by insuring that proper techniques are utilized in performing the measurements required.

    Despite all precautions, errors in measurement will occur. Small random fluctuations cannot be eliminated. They are due to chance breezes, to local (minor) temperature changes, to limits in human vision, to accidental vibrations, and to whims of providence, among other causes. Since these deviations are random, they may be either positive or negative.

    Which of the following errors are systematic? Which are random?

A. A balance is used to find the weight of some tablets. One of the 10-g weights has been chipped, and the recorded weight of the tablets is too high.
B. A pharmacist checks the rest point of a balance. The pointer indicates a reading of zero. A moment later, she checks it again. The pointer is slightly to the left. When she checks it again, the pointer is slightly to the right of zero.
C. A pharmacist uses a transfer pipet to measure out 1 mL of a liquid. Then he mistakenly blows through it to get out the last few drops. The volume delivered exceeds 1 mL.

- -

B is a random error and probably cannot be eliminated. A and C are systematic. The error in A can be detected by checking the weights in the set against each other. The error in C can be eliminated by use of proper technique.

---

31. Each measurement is an estimate of true value. However, our information is incomplete unless we have some notion of the amount of error involved. Without knowing what magnitude of deviation to anticipate, it is difficult to decide the degree of confidence to put in the measured quantity.

    To adequately specify a measured quantity, the two elements required are

- -

Estimate of true value; indication of error

32. When working with large quantities of data, as does the sociologist interested in smokers' habits or the pharmacologist concerned about the effect of a drug on the reproductive capacity of rats, the results are analyzed statistically. The mean, or perhaps the median, becomes the estimate of "true value," and the standard deviation may be employed as a measure of dispersion or deviation. However, in compounding prescriptions or weighing materials for manufacturing, pharmacists usually perform only a single measurement on each material handled. They are thus unable to make use of these statistical tools and must designate experimental quantities in other ways.

   If we know that determination of the weight of a sample of powder is subject to a maximum error of 10 mg, a 450-mg sample could be indicated as 450 mg ± 10 mg. We are therefore stating that the actual weight is approximately 450 mg and that it lies somewhere between 440 and 460 mg. Thus one way to indicate a measured quantity is to submit an estimate of true value and state the maximum deviation explicitly.

A. The volume of a sample of liquid is stated to be 27.0 ± 0.5 mL. Between what limits does the true volume fall?
B. A tablet is required to contain 45 to 55 mg of active ingredient. Express this requirement in terms of a desired weight and maximum error.

_____

A. 26.5 to 27.5 mL
B. 50 ± 5 mg

_____

33. A liquid product is required to have a specific gravity of 0.904 ± 0.012. Three batches of the liquid product are manufactured and their specific gravities are:

   Batch 1: 0.920
   Batch 2: 0.911
   Batch 3: 0.893

Which batches fall within the specific gravity requirement? Which do not?

_____

Batch 1 does not meet the standard because its specific gravity differs from 0.904 by a value greater than 0.012. Batch 2 and batch 3 pass this test.

---

34. Another way to indicate accuracy is to write the limit of error as a percentage of estimated value. Instead of writing 30 g ± 3 g, this quantity could be expressed as 30 g ± 10%, since 3 g are 10% of 30 g. Thus, 400 g ± 5% means 400 g ± 5% of 400 g. What is 5% of 400 g?

_ _

20 g

(If you had difficulty or would like to review percentage calculations, go to the next frame. Otherwise, go on to frame 36.)

---

35. The easiest way to handle percentage problems is first to convert percent to a decimal. This is accomplished by moving the decimal point two places to the left:

35% = 0.35

0.02% = 0.0002

To find the value of the percent of a quantity, change the percent to a decimal and multiply by the quantity.

13% of 40 tons = 0.13 × 40 tons = 5.2 tons.

1.5% of 12 g = 0.015 × 12 g = 0.18 g

To find the percent of a quantity represented by some component value, divide that value by the total quantity and move the decimal point two places to the right. Make sure that the units are the same. For example, 3 oz are what percent of 15 oz?

$$\frac{3 \text{ oz}}{15 \text{ oz}} = 0.2 = 20\%$$

What percent of 120 mg are 6 mg?

$$\frac{6 \text{ mg}}{120 \text{ mg}} = 0.05 = 5\%$$

Now try these problems. In A, B and C, convert the percentages shown to decimals.

A.   12.3% =
B.   0.175% =
C.   141% =
D.   Find 6% of 50 gal

E.   What is 25% of 14 hours?

F.   Find 1/2% of 200 lb.

What percent of 80 g are the following?
G.   32 g
H.   0.04 g

_____

A.   0.123
B.   0.00175
C.   1.41
D. 0.06×50 gal = 3 gal
E. 0.25×14 h = 3.5 h
F.   1/2% = 0.5% = 0.005; 0.005×200 lb = 1 lb

G. $\dfrac{32 \text{ g}}{80 \text{ g}} = 0.4 = 40\%$

H. $\dfrac{0.04 \text{ g}}{80 \text{ g}} = 0.0005 = 0.05\%$

36. Since 5% of 400 g is 20 g, 400 g ± 5% means 400 g ± 20 g. The actual value falls between 380 and 420 g. The standard for a particular type of drug might require that tablets contain 95 to 105% of the labeled amount of drug. This is another way of stating "labeled amount ± 5%," so that a tablet that is supposed to contain 200 mg of the drug may actually contain 200 mg ± 5%, or anywhere between 190 and 210 mg, and still be acceptable.

A. An industrial pharmacist must weigh 12.00 kg of a chemical. If a deviation of 2% is permissible, within what limits must the weighed quantity fall?

B. A hospital pharmacist must measure 19 to 21 mL of a liquid for a formula. Express this volume as a desired quantity with a maximum percent error.

_ _

A. Since 2% of 12.00 kg is 0.24 kg, the weight may be written as 12.00 kg ± 0.24 kg. The limits are therefore 11.76 to 12.24 kg.

B. 20 mL ± 5%

---

37. Try these problems:

A. The temperature inside a reaction vessel in a manufacturing plant is supposed to be 225°C ± 8%. If the actual temperature is 202°C is this acceptable?

B. The standard set by a manufacturer for a particular product states that each tablet must contain 95 to 105% of the labeled amount of drug. If the labeled amount of drug is 80 mg, what is the largest amount of drug that the tablet may contain if it is to be considered acceptable?

A. No. 8% of 225 is 18. The lowest permissible temperature is 207°C.

B. 84 mg

---

38. In many cases, measured weights and volumes are not written so as to indicate explicitly the maximum error incurred. However, the accuracy of the determination is implied by the number of figures used in its expression. The last figure written is always approximate. For example, the volume 70.8 mL implies that the "8" is uncertain. The true volume falls between 70.75 and 70.85 mL. In other words, 70.8 mL is accurate to the nearest 0.1 mL. Consider the following ways of writing the volume:

70.8 mL = 70.8 mL ± 0.05 mL
   (accurate to nearest 0.1 mL)

70.80 mL = 70.80 mL ± 0.005 mL
   (accurate to nearest 0.01 mL)

70.800 mL = 70.800 mL ± 0.0005 mL
   (accurate to nearest 0.001 mL)

Here, 70.8 mL, 70.80 mL, and 70.800 mL all indicate the same estimate of volume, but with a different degree of accuracy implied in each case. By using this convention of *significant figures*, the way in which a measured quantity is written provides an indication of both true value and measurement accuracy.

A. If an object is said to weigh 37.38 g, between what limits is the actual weight expected to fall?

B. If a tablet's weight is recorded as 2.6 g, to how many grams is the measurement accurate?

A. 37.38 ± 0.005 g = 37.375 to 37.385 g

B. 2.6 g = 2.6 g ± 0.05 g, accurate to the nearest 0.1 g

---

39. A capsule is weighed on a triple beam balance, which is accurate to the nearest 0.1 g. The balance riders indicate exactly twelve grams and the weight is recorded as 12.000 g. Is this designation correct?

No. Writing 12.000 g means that the measurement was accurate to the nearest 0.001 g. This implies a greater degree of accuracy than was achieved. The weight should have been recorded as 12.0 g.

40. If a tablet, placed on a balance accurate to the nearest 0.01 g, has a weight of exactly two grams, how should this value be written?

_ _

2.00 g. More zeros would imply a higher degree of accuracy than the balance is capable of. Fewer zeros would imply less accuracy than was actually obtained.

41. The thickness of a section of frog skin is recorded as 0.014 cm. The device used to make the measurement must have been accurate to the nearest

A. cm
B. 0.1 cm
C. 0.01 cm
D. 0.001 cm
E. 0.0001 cm
F. It is impossible to tell.

_ _

D is correct. Writing 0.014 cm means that the actual value falls between 0.0135 and 0.0145 cm and is accurate to the nearest 0.001 cm.

42. Each digit that is part of an experimental value, including the single uncertain digit, is significant. Zeros are significant unless they are included only to locate the decimal point.
    For each of the following measured quantities, determine the number of significant figures:

A. 4.73 g
B. 4.730 g
C. 0.0065 kg
D. 6500 kg

_ _

A. 3
B. 4. The final zero is not needed to fix the decimal point. It is included to indicate the degree of accuracy.

C.   2. The zeros locate the decimal point and are not really part of the measured value. The quantity could have been written 6.5 g, which clearly has two significant figures.

D.   2, 3, or 4. It is impossible to tell whether the zeros are significant or merely locate the decimal point. All ambiguity would be removed by using power-of-10 notation. Thus, if the weight were written 6.5×10^3 kg, we would see that it had two significant figures. If written 6.50×10^3 kg, the quantity would have three significant figures, since the zero is not needed to locate the decimal point.

43.   One cannot take a relatively inaccurate weight or volume and make it more exact by performing some calculation or transformation. The only way to reduce uncertainty is to use a more accurate instrument or technique. As a consequence, we must be careful that the result of a calculation is not represented as being more accurate than the measurement(s) on which the calculation is based. The result is permitted to contain only one uncertain figure.

The following rules determine the way in which a calculation based on measured quantities should be written.

(1) When measured quantities are added or subtracted, the result can have no more *decimal places* than the measurement with the smallest number of decimal places.

(2) In multiplication or division involving experimental values, the final result can have no more *significant figures* than does the measurement with the smallest number of significant figures.

A.   0.20 mL of an oil is dissolved in enough alcohol to make 12.000 mL of a solution. Calculate the amount of oil in each milliliter of the solution, paying attention to the number of significant figures.

B.   A foot powder contains two ingredients; each was weighed on a different balance with different accuracy. The powder contains 1.003 g of ingredient A and 35.4 g of ingredient B. Estimate the total weight of the foot powder.

A. 0.017 mL. The experimental value with the smallest number of significant figures, 0.20, has two figures. The result must also have two significant figures.

B. 36.4 g. In addition or subtraction involving experimental quantities, the result should contain no more decimal places than the quantity with the fewest decimal places. The simplest way to handle such a calculation is to carry it out to one decimal place more than that of the quantity with fewest places and then round off.

---

44. All of the examples in the preceding frames have dealt with situations in which calculations were performed using experimentally determined quantities. In those instances, the accuracy of the calculated result depended on the accuracy of the measurements made previous to the calculation.

   In prescription compounding or pharmaceutical manufacturing, the quantity of a particular ingredient that is to be weighed or measured is specified by a formula or is calculated from it. In either case, the accuracy to which the measurement must be made is not determined by the number of significant figures that happen to appear in the formula quantity. Its accuracy is determined by the nature of the end product and the manipulative processes that will be employed. Tolerances permitted in prescription compounding are generally larger than those allowed in industrial pharmacy.

   A formula for morphine sulfate tablets directs that 5 g of morphine sulfate be weighed. Does this mean that a balance accurate to the nearest gram may be used, since the formula quantity has only one significant figure?

Absolutely not! The maximum permissible error in weighing is not determined by the number of significant figures in the formula.

---

45. As a general rule, the maximum tolerable error in weighing or measuring a sample for prescription compounding is 5%. If a prescription formula calls for 0.5 g of ammonium chloride the pharmacist is obliged to weigh the ammonium chloride so as to

incur an error of no more than 5%. The balance used must be accurate enough so that the maximum error is 0.025 g.

A prescription requires 0.8 mL of glycerin and 30.00 mL of alcohol. What is the maximum error, in milliliters, that is permissible in measuring each of these liquids?

_ _

Glycerin: 5% of 0.8 mL = 0.04 mL
Alcohol: 5% of 30.00 mL = 1.5 mL

The tolerance in measurement does not depend on the number of significant figures in the formula.

46. The instrument usually used by the pharmacist for liquid volume measurement is the graduate. Graduates may be cylindrical or conical in shape. The error incurred in using a conical graduate depends on the volume measured. With a cylindrical graduate, the magnitude of the error is independent of the volume. But the percent error is not constant. It does depend on the volume that is being measured in the graduate.

For example, let us say that we are using a 100-mL graduated cylinder in which the error in reading the graduations is 1.0 mL. If 100 mL are measured, the percent error may be found by dividing the magnitude of the error by the actual volume.

1.0 mL/100 mL = 0.01 = 1%

If 50 mL are measured, 1.0 mL/50 mL = 0.02 = 2%.

What is the percent error if 20 mL are measured in the same graduate?

_ _

5%

Solution:

1.0 mL/20 mL = 0.05 = 5%

---

47. As the volume measured in a cylindrical graduate becomes smaller, the percent error

A. increases
B. decreases
C. remains the same

—————————————————

A is correct. This is apparent from our calculations in frame 46.

---

48. The pharmacist generally has an assortment of graduates of various sizes. To measure a given quantity of liquid, choose a graduate that will be filled as close to capacity as possible, to minimize the percent error. This is true for conical graduates as well, although in these graduates the error is a function of the volume of liquid measured. No graduate should be used to measure a volume that is less than 20% of its capacity.

   The smallest graduate commonly found in the pharmacy has a capacity of 10 mL. What is the smallest quantity that should be measured in this graduate?

—————————————————

2.0 mL. If less than 2.0 mL is to be measured, the pharmacist must resort to another type of instrument, such as a pipet or buret. It is also possible to use a calibrated dropper to measure small volumes, as we shall see later.

---

49. The balance used in weighing drugs for prescription compounding is a fairly sensitive instrument. In a balance that meets current standards, the sensitivity requirement is 6 mg. This means that a load of 6 mg causes a deflection of at least one scale division of the pointer. The balance is therefore capable of discriminating a minimum difference of 6 mg. This amount represents the maximum error in weighing that will be incurred using a prescription balance in proper working order.

   Table 1–1 shows how the maximum percent error changes depending on the amount that is weighed. Since the maximum percent error that is acceptable in weighing for prescription compounding is 5%, we see that it is all right to use the prescription balance to weigh 1500 mg or 150 mg but that the percent error involved in weighing 15 mg is much too great. Just as with the cylindrical graduate, the percent error increases as the amount weighed becomes smaller. From these data, we can tell that somewhere between 150 mg and 15 mg a particular quantity exists such that the error in weighing would be exactly 5%. That quantity is the smallest amount that can be weighed on a prescription balance with acceptable accuracy.

Table 1–1. Effect of Amount Weighed on Percent Error

Amount Weighed (mg)	Error (mg)	% Error
1500	6	0.4
150	6	4
15	6	40

Calculate the minimum weighable quantity for a prescription balance with a sensitivity requirement of 6 mg.

_____

120 mg

Solution:

Let j equal minimum weighable quantity:

$$0.05 = \frac{6 \text{ mg}}{j}$$

j = 120 mg

This calculation shows that if a quantity of 120 mg or more is weighed on a prescription balance, the error will be 5% or less. The accuracy will therefore be acceptable. If less than 120 mg of a drug is required, direct weighing of that quantity on a prescription balance will lead to unacceptably large errors. Other techniques must be used. These will be introduced later in the book.

50. A. What is the maximum percent error incurred if a balance
        with a sensitivity requirement of 15 mg is used to weigh 120
        mg of a powder?
    B. What is the minimum weighable quantity with a maximum
        error of 5% on a balance whose sensitivity requirement is 30
        mg?

- -

A. 12.5%
B. 600 mg

Solutions:

A. 15 mg/120 mg = 0.125 = 12.5%
B. Let j equal minimum weighable quantity:

$$0.05 = \frac{30 \text{ mg}}{j}$$

$j = 600$ mg

---

51. In pharmaceutical manufacturing, tolerances in measurement
    are more stringent than in prescription compounding.
    Manufacturing involves larger quantities, more manipulation,
    and use of more complicated techniques than does compounding.
    Each operation provides an opportunity for error. Although the
    errors may each be small, they may be additive, leading to an
    unacceptable product. There is no generally accepted standard for
    measurement accuracy in industrial practice similar to the
    guideline for prescription compounding, but certainly the
    maximum error in weighing or measuring should be less than
    1%.

A. The maximum percent error in measurement for prescription
    compounding is _____ .
B. The maximum percent error in measurement for
    pharmaceutical manufacturing is _____ .

- -

A. 5%

B.   Less than 1%

52. What is the smallest quantity that can be weighed with 1% maximum error on a balance whose sensitivity requirement is 1.0 mg?

_ _

100 mg

Solution:

Let j equal minimum weighable quantity:

$$\frac{1 \text{ mg}}{j} = 0.01$$

$$j = 100 \text{ mg}$$

53. Here are some problems that review the material covered in this chapter. Do not look at the answers until you have finished all of them. Remember to use estimation to ensure that the decimal point is placed where it belongs

A. $4670 = 4.67 \times 10$?

B. $0.04589 = 4.589 \times 10$?

C. $8.91 \times 10^3 = ?$

D. $12.8 \times 10^{-6} = ?$

E.   Two feet of wire weigh 9.09 g. How many inches would weigh 170 g?

F. If 3.00 g of an ointment contain 4.25×10^3 units of vitamin A, how many grams would contain 500 units?

G. An acre is 43,560 ft². If land is taxed at $150 per acre, calculate the tax to the nearest dollar on a rectangular piece of land that is 200 ft by 300 ft.

H. If there are 737 peanuts to a pound and they cost 90¢ per quarter-pound, how many peanuts can you buy for $1.75?

I. If a formula calls for 36 g of a drug to make 80,000 tablets, how many grams will each tablet contain?

J. If 1 joule = 0.24 calorie and 1 calorie = 1.16×10^{-6} kilowatt-hours, how many kilowatt-hours are equivalent to 1500 joules?

K. A certain tablet is required to contain 90 to 110% of the labeled amount of active ingredient. Between what limits (in milligrams) must the amount of drug in a 200-mg tablet fall?

L. If the error in using a balance is 10 mg, what would the percent error be if 300 mg were weighed?

M. A tablet is required to contain 46 to 54 mg of active ingredient. Express this requirement as a desired quantity and maximum percent error.

N. How many significant figures are there in each of the quantities that follow:

(1) 0.035 g
(2) 0.350 g
(3) 427.2 kg

O. In the two examples that follow, an arithmetic operation is to be performed on quantities that have been measured. Make certain that your answers contain the correct number of figures.

(1) The amount of liquid in a bottle is measured in a graduated cylinder and found to be 172 mL. On separate occasions, using a pipet, the following quantities are withdrawn: 12.00 mL, 3.75 mL and 1.008 mL. Calculate the amount remaining in the bottle.

(2) Using a mold, 0.94 g of a drug is used to make six suppositories. How much of the drug is contained in each suppository? (A quantity that can easily be counted, such as six suppositories, is taken to be an absolute, not an approximate, quantity and so is not subject to measurement error.)

P.   One of the components in a prescription formula is sodium chloride, 1.2 g. Between what limits must the actual weight fall in order to meet the usual standard of accuracy?

Q.   A formula for 100,000 tablets requires 400 mg of a potent drug. Between what limits must the actual weight of the drug fall if the maximum permissible error in weighing is 0.5%?

R.   What is the smallest quantity that should be measured using a 120-mL conical graduate?

S.   What is the smallest quantity that can be weighed on a prescription balance (with a sensitivity requirement of 6 mg) with a maximum error of 2%?

T. What maximum percent error is anticipated if 450 mg of powder are weighed on a balance whose sensitivity requirement is 18 mg?

U. What is the smallest quantity that can be weighed with a maximum error of 1% on a balance whose sensitivity requirement is 0.1 g?

V. What is the smallest volume that can be measured with acceptable accuracy for prescription compounding in a 2-mL pipet in which the maximum error is 0.005 mL, independent of the volume measured?

_____

A. 4.67×10^3
B. 4.589×10^{-2}
C. 8910
D. 0.0000128
E. 449 in.
F. 0.353 g
G. $207
H. 358
I. 4.5×10^{-4} g
J. 4.2×10^{-4} kilowatt-hours
K. 180 to 220 mg
L. 3.3%
M. 50 mg ± 4 mg or 50 mg ± 8%
N. (1) 2
    (2) 3
    (3) 4

O. (1) 155 mL. The original measurement of the contents of the bottle was accurate to the nearest milliliter, so a sum or difference involving that quantity can only be accurate to the nearest milliliter.

(2) 0.16 g. When dividing measured quantities, the result can have no more significant figures than the component with the fewest significant figures.

P. A maximum tolerance of 5% is permitted: 1.14 to 1.26 g

Q. 398 to 402 mg

R. 20% of 120 mL = 24 mL

S. 300 mg

T. 4%

U. 10 g

V. 0.1 mL

CHAPTER TWO

UNITS AND CONVERSION

Although the metric system has not been generally adopted in the United States, all units of pharmaceutical measurement are defined in terms of metric standards. The *United States Pharmacopeia* (USP) and other compendia of drug specifications and product formulas use only the metric system, and essentially all prescription and hospital medication orders are written in terms of metric units. Two other systems require brief mention. The apothecary system, once widely used in prescription writing, is now largely of historical interest, but some units and symbols survive to this day. The avoirdupois system is still used in commerce in the United States. Typically, the capacity of containers for pharmaceutical products is described in terms of ounces.

After reviewing the various systems in this chapter, we explore the relationships that allow switching units from one system to another.

Learning objectives: after completing this chapter the student should be able to

1. Name the metric units for weight, volume and length and state the relationships within each group of units.
2. List the most important apothecary and avoirdupois units.
3. Convert quantities from metric units to apothecary and avoirdupois units, and vice versa.

1. The standard unit of mass in the metric system is the kilogram (kg). The gram (g) is defined in terms of the kilogram:

$$1 \text{ g} = 0.001 \text{ kg} = 10^{-3} \text{ kg}$$

or

$$1 \text{ kg} = 1000 \text{ g} = 10^3 \text{ g}$$

These equations allow us to convert from one unit to the other.

A. Express 0.370 kg in terms of grams.

B. Express 11.2 g in terms of kilograms.

_____

A. 0.370 kg = 370 g

B. 11.2 g = 0.0112 kg

---

2. The following list provides relationships between the pharmaceutically important metric units of mass:

$$1 \text{ kg} = 1000 \text{ g} = 10^3 \text{ g}$$

$$1 \text{ g} = 1000 \text{ milligrams (mg)} = 10^3 \text{ mg}$$

$$1 \text{ mg} = 1000 \text{ micrograms (µg or mcg)} = 10^3 \text{ µg}$$

$$1 \text{ µg} = 1000 \text{ nanograms (ng)} = 10^3 \text{ ng}$$

$$1 \text{ g} = 10^{-3} \text{ kg} = 10^3 \text{ mg} = 10^6 \text{ µg} = 10^9 \text{ ng}$$

Review these relationships. When you are familiar with them, fill in the blanks.

A. 1 mg = _____ g = _____ kg = _____ µg = _____ ng
B. 1 kg = _____ g = _____ mg = _____ µg
C. 1 g = _____ µg = _____ mg = _____ ng = _____ kg

_____

A. 1 mg = 0.001 g (10^{-3} g) = 0.000001 kg (10^{-6} kg) = 1000 µg (10^3 µg) = 1,000,000 ng (10^6 ng)
B. 1 kg = 1000 g (10^3 g) = 1,000,000 mg (10^6 mg) = 1,000,000,000 µg (10^9 µg)
C. 1 g = 1,000,000 µg (10^6 µg) = 1000 mg (10^3 mg) = 1,000,000,000 ng (10^9 ng) = 0.001 kg (10^{-3} kg)

(If you got these right, move on; if not, review and try again.)

---

3. Fill in the blanks:

A. 1275 mg =   g

B. 130 mg =   μg

C. 0.032 g =   mg

D. 455 mg =   kg

E. 0.0075 g =   μg

F. 0.030 mg =   g

G. 8.8×10^5 μg =   kg

H. 0.094 kg =   g

I. 62 ng =   mg

A. 1.275 g
B. 130,000 μg (or 1.3×10^5 μg)
C. 32 mg
D. 0.000455 kg (or 4.55×10^{-4} kg)
E. 7500 μg
F. 0.000030 g (or 3.0×10^{-5} g)
G. 8.8×10^{-4} kg
H. 94 g
I. 6.2×10^{-5} mg

(If you had a perfect score, proceed to the next frame. If you had trouble setting up your conversions, review Chapter 1. If you attempted the problems before learning the table, go back and study it. Do not go on to the next frame until you can do every problem in this frame correctly.)

---

4. The following listing describes the metric units most frequently used by pharmacists in measuring volume:

   1 liter (L) = 1000 milliliters (mL) = 10^3 mL

   1 mL = 1000 microliters (μL) = 10^3 μL

   1 mL = 1 cubic centimeter (cc)

$$1 \text{ L} = 10^3 \text{ mL} = 10^3 \text{ cc} = 10^6 \text{ μL}$$

When you have learned the above, fill in the blanks:

A.   1 mL = _____ cc = _____ L = _____ μL

B.   1 L = _____ μL = _____ cc

C.   1 μL = _____ mL = _____ L

- -

    A.   1 mL = 1 cc = 0.001 L (10^{-3} L) = 1000 μL (10^3 μL)
    B.   1 L = 1,000,000 μL (10^6 μL) = 1000 cc (10^3 cc)
    C.   1 μL = 0.001 mL = 10^{-6} L

(If you were right, go to the next frame. Otherwise, review the table.)

---

5.   Fill in the blanks:

A.   2.6 mL =   cc

B.   3.5 L =   cc

C.   0.4 mL =   μL

D.   0.1 μL =   L

E.   6 mL =   L

F.   2.37 L =   mL

G.   0.072 cc =   μL

- -

    A.   2.6 cc
    B.   3500 cc = 3.5×10^3 cc
    C.   400 μL
    D.   0.0000001 L = 1×10^{-7} L
    E.   0.006 L = 6×10^{-3} L
    F.   2370 mL = 2.37×10^3 mL
    G.   72 μL

(If you had a perfect score, proceed to frame 6. If you ran into trouble, review now to overcome any difficulties. Do not proceed to the next frame until you can do every problem in this frame correctly.)

6. The metric units of length most frequently encountered by pharmacists are as follows:

$$1 \text{ meter (m)} = 100 \text{ centimeters (cm)} = 10^2 \text{ cm}$$

$$1 \text{ m} = 1000 \text{ millimeters (mm)} = 10^3 \text{ mm}$$

$$1 \text{ mm} = 1000 \text{ micrometers (μm)} = 10^3 \text{ μm}$$

$$1 \text{ μm} = 1000 \text{ nanometers (nm)} = 10^3 \text{ nm}$$

$$1 \text{ m} = 10^2 \text{ cm} = 10^3 \text{ mm} = 10^6 \text{ μm} = 10^9 \text{ nm}$$

When you are familiar with the above, do these problems:

A. 170 cm =   mm
B. 12.5 μm =   mm
C. 0.2 cm =   m
D. 0.32 m =   mm
E. 0.013 m =   cm
F. 744 μm =   cm
G. 6.19 mm =   nm
H. 0.08 m =   μm

————————————————————

A. 1700 mm
B. 0.0125 mm
C. 0.002 m = 2×10^{-3} m
D. 320 mm
E. 1.3 cm
F. 0.0744 cm
G. 6.19×10^6 nm
H. 8×10^4 μm

(If you had a perfect score, proceed to frame 8. If not, be sure you understand how to do each problem before going any further.)

7. The following problems review the material covered in the preceding frames. If you were able to get all of the problems in frames 3 to 7 right on the first try, you may, if you wish, go directly to frame 9.

A. 470 μL =   mL
B. 0.095 g =   mg
C. 1.5 L =   cc
D. 340 mm =   m
E. 2500 μg =   mg

F.   870 g =   kg
G. 3.7×10^4 mL =   L
H.   235 μm =   cm
I.   32 cc =   mL
J.   0.055 g =   μg
K.   57 mg =   kg
L.   42.2 μL =   L
M.   0.003 kg =   μg
N.   12.3 m =   cm
O.   958 μm =   mm
P.   78.3 μL =   cc
Q.   14 cm =   mm
R.   0.082 mg =   ng

_____

A.   0.47 mL
B.   95 mg
C.   1500 cc
D.   0.34 m
E.   2.5 mg
F.   0.87 kg
G.   37 L
H.   0.0235 cm
I.   32 mL
J. 5.5×10^4 μg (55,000 μg)
K. 5.7×10^{-5} kg
L. 4.22×10^{-5}
M. 3×10^6 μg
N.   1230 cm
O.   0.958 mm
P.   0.0783 cc
Q.   140 mm
R.   82,000 ng

8.   A pharmacist, on separate occasions, dispenses 220 mg and 450 mg of a certain drug. How much of the drug remains if the bottle originally contained 1.50 g? (Remember to estimate the result in this problem and those that follow as a check.)

_____

830 mg or 0.83 g

Solution:

Before adding or subtracting quantities, they must be expressed in the same units.

220 mg + 450 mg = 670 mg = 0.67 g (total dispensed)

1.50 g − 0.67 g = 0.83 g (remainder)

---

9. A patient receives 500 μg of estradiol benzoate by injection every day for 22 days. How many grams of estradiol benzoate does the patient receive altogether?

_____

0.011 g

Solution:

The total amount administered is equal to the product of the daily dose and the number of days.

500 μg/day × 22 days = 11,000 μg = 11 mg = 0.011 g

---

10. If 25.0 mL of an oil are used in the manufacture of 125,000 capsules, how many microliters of oil are contained in each capsule?

_____

0.200 μL

Solution:

$$\frac{25 \text{ mL}}{125,000 \text{ caps}} = 2.00 \times 10^{-4} \text{ mL/caps} = 0.200 \text{ µL/caps}$$

---

11. A solution contains 125 mg of a drug in each milliliter. How many milliliters contain 2.50 g of the drug?

- -

20.0 mL

Solution:

$$2.5 \text{ g} = 2500 \text{ mg}; \quad \frac{125 \text{ mg}}{1 \text{ mL}} = \frac{2500 \text{ mg}}{j}$$

$$j = 20.0 \text{ mL}$$

---

12. Do all of the problems in this frame before verifying any of the answers. Work carefully using an estimate as a check. Write all units down, and make certain that the units in your final solution are consistent with the quantities that enter into the calculation.

A. In 25.0 mL of a solution for injection there are 4.00 mg of the drug. If the dose to be administered to a patient is 200 µg, what quantity of this solution should be used?

B. A patient is to be given capsules, each containing 22.0 mg of hydrocortisone. How many grams of hydrocortisone are required to make 60 such capsules?

C. If 0.50 L of a medicinal solution is dispensed to a patient who takes 1 tablespoonful of the solution four times a day for seven full days, how many milliliters of the solution remain? (1 tablespoonful equals 15 mL.)

D. A capsule contains 4 µg of a potent drug. How many capsules could be made from 0.332 kg of the drug?

E. How many liters of a solution are needed to fill 250 bottles, each containing 45.0 cc of the solution?

F. If 3.17 kg of a drug are used to make 50,000 tablets, how many milligrams will 30 tablets contain?

G. A medicated disk has a thickness of 4.80 mm. What would be the height, in centimeters, of a stack of 24 medicated disks?

H. How many microliters of oil does each glass vial contain if 2.1 L of the oil were used to uniformly fill 6×10^4 glass vials?

I.   If 0.625 kg of a drug is used to make 250,000 tablets, how many tablets contain 0.125 g?

- -

A.   1.25 mL
B.   1.32 g
C.   80 mL
D. $83 \times 10^6 = 83,000,000$ capsules
E.   11.3 L
F.   1900 mg
G.   11.5 cm
H.   35 μL
I.   50 tablets

(If any of your answers do not agree with these, read the problem(s) again and check your calculations. If you still have trouble, study the full solutions below. To review the units of this system, go back to frame 3. To review the techniques used in problem solving, go back to the first chapter. It is important that you clear things up now, before we leave the metric system.)

Solutions:

A. $\dfrac{4000\ \text{μg}}{25\ \text{mL}} = \dfrac{200\ \text{μg}}{j}$

$j = 1.25$ mL

Estimate: by inspection, j is 1/20 of 25 mL or about 1 mL

B.   22.0 mg/caps $\times$ 60 caps $\times \dfrac{1\ \text{g}}{1000\ \text{mg}} = 1.32$ g

C.   The patient has taken a total of 28 tablespoonfuls. Since 1 tablespoonful = 15 mL, he has taken 28 tablespoonfuls $\times$ 15 mL/tablespoonful = 420 mL.

500 mL − 420 mL = 80 mL

D. $0.332 \text{ kg} = 332 \text{ g} = 332 \times 10^6 \text{ µg}$

$$\frac{332 \times 10^6 \text{ µg}}{4 \text{ µg/caps}} = 83 \times 10^6 \text{ capsules}$$

E. $45.0 \text{ cc/bottle} \times 250 \text{ bottles} = 11,300 \text{ cc} = 11.3 \text{ L}$

F. $3.17 \text{ kg} = 3.17 \times 10^6 \text{ mg}$

$$\frac{3.17 \times 10^6 \text{ mg}}{5 \times 10^4 \text{ tablets}} = \frac{j}{30 \text{ tablets}}$$

$j = 1900 \text{ mg}$

(Only three significant figures should be written because the weight of the drug was accurate to three figures.)

G. $4.80 \text{ mm} \times 24 = 115 \text{ mm} = 11.5 \text{ cm}$

H. $2.1 \text{ L} = 2.1 \times 10^6 \text{ µL}$

$$\frac{2.1 \times 10^6 \text{ µL}}{6 \times 10^4 \text{ vials}} = 35 \text{ µL/vial}$$

I. $$\frac{625 \text{ g}}{2.5 \times 10^5 \text{ tablets}} = \frac{0.125 \text{ g}}{j}$$

$j = 50 \text{ tablets}$

---

13. Another system of units formerly employed in prescription writing is the apothecary system. The basic unit of apothecary weight is the grain (gr). Be careful not to confuse "gr" and "g". This is no problem when these units appear on a printed page, but be careful when reading handwritten prescriptions or performing calculations yourself. The gram is equivalent to about 15 gr, and transposition of one unit for the other could have serious consequences.

   The table that follows lists the apothecary weight units. Roman numerals are frequently used in connection with apothecary units, very often following the symbol for the unit rather than preceding it.

   20 gr = 1 scruple

   60 gr = 1 dram (1 ʒ, ʒ I)

   480 gr = 8 drams = 1 apothecary ounce (1 ℥)

Note that the apothecary ounce is different in magnitude from the avoirdupois (household) unit with the same name. This listing is provided for reference only; since the apothecary system has lost its importance, we will not do any calculations with these units. The only exception is the grain, which on rare occasions is still employed as an indicator of drug dosage.

---

14. The units used to indicate apothecary fluid measure are identical to those used for common fluid measure in the United States. They are given below.

   60 minims = 1 fluidram (1 f₃ or f₃ I)

   8 f₃ = 1 fluidounce (1 f℥ or f℥ I)

   16 f℥ = 1 pint (1 pt)

   2 pt = 1 qt

   4 qt = 1 gallon (1 gal, 1 Cong, or 1 C)

   This system of fluid measure is important largely because most packages are still manufactured with capacities quoted in ounces rather than metric units. Thus, if the pharmacist prepares 30 mL of a liquid medication, that product would be put into a 1-fluidounce container. The minim and fluidram are no longer used for prescription measurements. However, the symbol for the fluidram survives as a way of writing "teaspoonful" on prescription orders. We'll come back to this point in Chapter 5.
   Review the symbols and abbreviations of these units and the relationships between them. When you have learned them, try these questions.

A. Write the full name of each unit.

   (1) Cong
   (2) f℥
   (3) gal
   (4) pt
   (5) f₃

B. Write the symbol or abbreviation for each unit.

   (1) fluidounce
   (2) gallon
   (3) fluidram
   (4) pint
   (5) quart

_____

A. (1) gallon
    (2) fluidounce
    (3) gallon
    (4) pint
    (5) fluidram

B. (1) f$\mathfrak{Z}$
    (2) gal, Cong, or C
    (3) f$\mathfrak{z}$
    (4) pt
    (5) qt

---

15. Complete these relations:

A. 1 qt =   pt
B. 1 f$\mathfrak{Z}$ =   f$\mathfrak{z}$
C. 1 gal =   qt
D. 1 pt =   f$\mathfrak{Z}$
E. 128 f$\mathfrak{Z}$ =   gal
F. 1 qt =   f$\mathfrak{Z}$
G. 2 gal =   pt

_____

A. 2 pt
B. 8 f$\mathfrak{z}$
C. 4 qt
D. 16 f$\mathfrak{Z}$
E. 1 gal
F. 32 f$\mathfrak{Z}$
G. 16 pt

(If you had a perfect score, go to frame 16. Otherwise, spend more time with this system of units and then try these questions once more.)

---

16. How many 3-f$\mathfrak{Z}$ bottles of cough syrup can be filled completely from a quart?

_____

10 full bottles

Solution:

$$\frac{32\ f\mathfrak{Z}}{3\ f\mathfrak{Z}/\text{bottle}} = 10 \text{ bottles } (2\ f\mathfrak{Z} \text{ remain unused})$$

---

17. A third system with which the pharmacist must be familiar is the avoirdupois system. The weight of articles shipped in commerce in the United States is usually given in avoirdupois weight. The avoirdupois system is not employed in prescription writing. In the avoirdupois system,

    437 1/2 grains = 1 ounce (1 oz)

    16 oz = 1 pound (1 lb)

    The apothecary grain and the avoirdupois grain are identical. But the "oz" and apothecary ounce are different.
    How many ounces are there in 1/2 lb?

_____

8

---

18. How many capsules, each containing 1/4 grain of phenobarbital, can be manufactured if a bottle containing 2 ounces of phenobarbital is available?

_____

3500 capsules

Solution:

$$2 \text{ oz} = 875 \text{ gr}; \frac{875 \text{ gr}}{0.25 \text{ gr/capsule}} = 3500 \text{ capsules}$$

19. These problems review the systems of units that are important in pharmacy practice. Use them to iron out any weak spots in your work.

A. How many milliliters of an oil are needed to prepare 640 capsules if 15 capsules contain 137 μL of the oil?

B. How many kilograms of sodium fluoride are needed to make 60,000 tablets of sodium fluoride tablets each containing 50 μg?

C. You have 15.8 g of tetracycline hydrochloride powder. How many 250-mg capsules can you make from this quantity of powder?

D. A nurse adds sufficient water to a vial containing 2 million units of penicillin to make a total volume of 5 mL of penicillin suspension. How many milliliters of the suspension should be injected into a child who is to receive a dose of 300,000 units?

E. A drug product contains 0.22 mL of an oil in each capsule. How many liters of the oil would be required for 4500 capsules?

F. How many tablets each containing 2.5 mg of amphetamine can be made from 0.620 kg of amphetamine?

G. How many micrograms of vitamin A are there in each tablet if 2.75 g of vitamin A are used to make 5000 tablets?

H. A manufacturer fills 490 bottles so that each bottle contains 30 mL of an oil. If he started with 15.5 L of the oil, how many milliliters are left after the filling operation is complete?

I. If 12.0 mg of a drug are present in 440 g of a powder, how many grams of drug would there be in 14.0 kg of powder?

- -

A. 5.85 mL
B. 0.003 kg
C. 63 capsules
D. 0.75 mL
E. 0.99 L
F. 2.48×10^5 tablets
G. 550 µg
H. 800 mL
I. 0.382 g

20. Despite the widespread utilization of the metric system, there are occasions when it is necessary to deal with quantities expressed in

other units. For example, these might be used to describe drug dosage (in grains) or a finished quantity of a prescription product (in ounces). In those cases, we will have to convert the values from one unit system to another.

The various systems have very different origins, and the relationships between units are usually not in terms of whole numbers. They are approximations expressed in enough significant figures to satisfy the particular application.

The United States Pharmacopoeia (<u>USP</u>) states that

1 g = 15.4324 gr

1 fluidounce = 29.5729 mL

These relations, referred to as *exact equivalents*, are actually highly refined approximations. They are used when pharmaceutical formulas for manufactured products are converted from one system to another. Conversions and other calculations for prescriptions do not require this high degree of accuracy. If a calculation is carried to three significant figures, the maximum error resulting from rounding is 0.5%. This is ample, considering that measurements for prescriptions are permitted a 5% tolerance. Consequently, for prescription compounding, the equivalents should be rounded to three significant figures:

1 g = 15.4 gr

1 fluidounce = 29.6 mL

According to the <u>USP</u>, 1 oz = 28.350 g. What conversion relationship should be used for

A.   prescription work?
B.   pharmaceutical manufacturing?

_____

A.   1 oz = 28.4 g
B.   1 oz = 28.350 g

---

21. Following is a collection of mathematical statements that allow conversion of weights among the metric, apothecary, and avoirdupois systems. They are given to three significant figures and are intended for use in prescription calculations.

1 g = 15.4 gr

1 oz = 28.4 g

1 gr (apothecary) = 1 gr (avoirdupois)

1 gr = 64.8 mg

1 kg = 2.20 lb

1 lb = 454 g

Only the first two expressions need be memorized, since all of the others may be derived from them. However, it's easy enough to memorize the others, thus reducing computation and saving time.

When you think you are sufficiently acquainted with the relationships, fill in the blanks.

A. 1 gr (avoirdupois) =   gr (apothecary)
B. 1 kg =   lb
C. 1 g =   gr
D. 1 gr =   mg
E. 1 lb =   g
F. 1 oz =   g

_____

A. 1 gr (apoth)
B. 2.20 lb
C. 15.4 gr
D. 64.8 mg
E. 454 g
F. 28.4 g

(You should have achieved a perfect score. If you did not, spend more time and try again.)

22. Remembering to estimate the result in each case, perform the following conversions using equivalency relationships to three significant figures:

A. 12 g =   gr

B. 12.4 lb =   kg

C. $\frac{1}{40}$ gr =   mg

D. 4 oz =   g

E. 2 lb =   g

_____

A. 185 gr
B. 5.64 kg
C. 1.62 mg
D. 114 g
E. 908 g

Since the conversion expressions all have three significant figures, so do the results.

---

23. Statements of equivalence that allow conversion of volume units include:

$$1 \, \text{f} \bar{\text{3}} = 29.6 \, \text{mL}$$

$$1 \, \text{pt} = 473 \, \text{mL}$$

Accuracy is to three figures, so these values are suitable for prescription calculations.
When you know these statements, fill in the blanks:

A. 1 f ʒ =   cc
B. 1 pt =   mL
C. 1 qt =   L

_____

A. 29.6 mL = 29.6 cc
B. 473 mL
C. 1 qt = 2 pt = 946 mL = 0.946 L

---

24. A medicinal syrup costs \$4.27 per pint. What is the cost of 45 mL?

_____

\$0.41

Solution:

$$\frac{\$4.27}{473 \, \text{mL}} = \frac{j}{45 \, \text{mL}}$$

$j = \$0.41$

---

25. By this point, you should be familiar with the following frequently used conversion relationships (with three significant figures).

A.   1 gr (apoth) =   gr (avoir)

B.   1 g =   gr

C.   1 f℥ =   mL

D.   1 gr =   mg

E.   1 kg =   lb

F.   1 oz =   g

G.   1 pt =   mL

- -

    A.   1
    B.   15.4
    C.   29.6
    D.   64.8
    E.   2.20
    F.   28.4
    G.   473

---

26. Here are some more problems that require conversion from one system of measurement to another. Use them for practice.

A.   How many milligrams of nitroglycerin are there in 60 tablets if each tablet contains 1/100 gr of nitroglycerin?

B.   Convert 1 qt to microliters.

C. If an ounce of papaverine costs $3.75, how many dollars would 146 gr cost?

D. Convert 60 g to grains.

E. Convert 6 f ℥ to milliliters.

F. If 1 lb of an ointment costs $6.30, what is the cost of 60 g of the ointment?

——————————————————

A. 38.9 mg
B. 9.46×10^5 μL
C. $1.25. The "ounce" was avoirdupois.
D. 924 gr
E. 178 mL
F. 83¢

27. Sometimes it will be necessary to convert several quantities to other unit systems. Here is an example.

A syrup contains 12.0 gr of a pain reliever in each fluidounce. How many milliliters contain 650 mg?

- -

24.7 mL

One way to attach this problem is first to find the number of milligrams per fluidounce and then use proportion to calculate the number of milliliters.

12.0 gr/fluidounce × 64.8 mg/gr = 778 mg/fluidounce

$$\frac{778 \text{ mg}}{29.6 \text{ mL}} = \frac{650 \text{ mg}}{j}$$

j = 24.7 mL

---

28. Try these for more practice:

A. Each fluidounce of cough syrup contains 1 gr of codeine. How many milligrams of codeine are present in 60 mL of the syrup?

B. If 1 pt of a syrup costs $16.25, what would be the cost of 50 mL?

- -

A. 131 mg
B. $1.72

---

29. A pharmacist receives a prescription for tablets containing aminophylline, 1 1/2 gr (which is equivalent to 97.2 mg). He has on hand aminophylline, 100 mg. What should he do?
    There is a table in the USP that lists *approximate equivalents*. The relationships given in that table are not to be used when

calculating quantities of materials that will be weighed or measured for a prescription. However, when a prefabricated dosage form (one prepared by a pharmaceutical manufacturer) is prescribed in one system of units but is available to the pharmacist in strengths given in a different system, it is permissible to dispense the strength that is approximately equivalent to that prescribed. Thus, it is permissible to dispense aminophylline tablets, 100 mg, when tablets are written for 1 1/2 gr. Some examples of approximate equivalents follow:

1 pt ≈ 500 mL

1 f ʒ ≈ 30 mL

1 gr ≈ 60 mg

1 1/2 gr ≈ 100 mg

1 ʒ ≈ 30 g

A.   A prescription calls for 500 mL of an antiseptic solution concentrate, but it is packaged in pints. What should the pharmacist do?

B.   A prescription specifies thyroid tablets, 1 gr. The pharmacist has a bottle of thyroid tablets, 60 mg. What should she do?

_ _

A.   Dispense a pint
B.   Dispense 60 mg tablets

No compounding or manufacturing is required in either case.

---

30.   Do all the problems in this frame before verifying your answers. Be certain to write units down and use them. Estimate your result or perform some other kind of check where possible.

A.   A formula for 48 capsules contains 125 gr of quinine. How many grams does each capsule contain?

B.   A pharmacist purchased 4 oz of sodium bromide for $3.50. What is the cost of 10 g?

C. The "average" adult weighs about 70 kg. How many pounds is this?

D. If 4 f℥ of a solution cost $1.25, what is the cost of 20 mL?

E. A pharmacist purchased 1 qt of a sterilizing solution and dispensed (on separate occasions) 1 pt and 250 mL. How many liters were left?

F. If a pint of a syrup costs $5.72, what will be the cost of 90.0 mL?

— — — — — — — — — — — — — — — — — —

A. 0.169 g
B. $0.31
C. 70 kg = 154 lb
D. $0.21
E. 0.223 L
F. $1.09

Solutions:

A. $125 \text{ gr} \times \dfrac{1 \text{ g}}{15.4 \text{ gr}} = 8.12 \text{ g}$

$\dfrac{8.12 \text{ g}}{48 \text{ caps}} = 0.169 \text{ g/caps}$

B. 4 oz cost \$3.50

$4 \text{ oz} \times 28.4 \text{ g/oz} = 114 \text{ g}$

$\dfrac{114 \text{ g}}{\$3.50} = \dfrac{10 \text{ g}}{j}$

$j = \$0.31$

C. $70 \text{ kg} \times 2.20 \text{ lb/kg} = 154 \text{ lb}$

D. $4 \text{ f} ʒ \times 29.6 \text{ mL/f} ʒ = 118 \text{ mL}$

$\dfrac{118 \text{ mL}}{\$ 1.25} = \dfrac{20 \text{ mL}}{j}$

$j = \$0.21$

E. 1 qt = 946 mL

dispensed: 473 mL + 250 mL = 723 mL

remaining: 946 mL − 723 mL = 223 mL = 0.223 L

F. $\dfrac{473 \text{ mL}}{\$5.72} = \dfrac{90.0 \text{ mL}}{j}$

$j = \$1.09$

CHAPTER THREE

OTHER EXAMPLES OF CONVERSION

Although weight and volume are the traditional ways of identifying the amount of drug, there are occasions when other measures are used. An example is potency units, used to standardize the activity of certain biologically derived drugs. Sometimes the relation between potency units and the amount of pure chemical is known so that it is possible to switch from one set of units to the other. Another situation that represents a kind of conversion is when a tablet or capsule serves as a source of drug. Sometimes, the weight of a liquid has to be calculated from its volume or, for convenience, volumetric measurement of a liquid is preferred when this substance is listed in a formula in terms of mass units. These examples of conversion are treated in this chapter.

Learning objectives: after completing this chapter the student should be able to

1. Calculate the number of tablets needed as a source of drug in prescription compounding.
2. Convert between potency units and weight units where a known relation exists.
3. Use the density to convert liquid volume to weight and vice versa.

---

1. A pharmacist needs hydrocortisone for a prescription but has this drug only in the form of tablets, each containing 20 mg. For these tablets, there is equivalence between the number of tablets and the quantity of drug. We may write

1 tablet = 20 mg hydrocortisone

A pharmacist needs 300 mg of hydrocortisone for a prescription. How many tablets, each containing 20 mg of hydrocortisone, will supply the quantity of drug required?

----

15 tablets

Solution:

$$300 \text{ mg} \times \frac{1 \text{ tablet}}{20 \text{ mg}} = 15 \text{ tablets}$$

Since each tablet contains 20 mg of hydrocortisone, the fraction in this expression equals unity. We are converting an expression of weight into one telling us the number of tablets that will deliver the needed weight of the drug.

2. A pharmacist receives a prescription requiring 4 mg of a drug. The drug is available in tablets, each of which contains 160 µg of active ingredient. How many tablets should be used?

----

25 tablets

Solution:

Conversion into the desired number of tablets is accomplished by realizing that

1 tablet = 160 µg = 0.16 mg

$$4 \text{ mg} \times \frac{1 \text{ tablet}}{0.16 \text{ mg}} = 25 \text{ tablets}$$

3. Here are two more problems involving conversion to tablets.

A. A prescription calls for 1.25 gr of Dilaudid. How many 3-mg tablets of Dilaudid should be used?

B. A prescription calls for 360 mg of a drug. How many 8-mg tablets of the drug will supply the needed quantity?

_____

A. 27 tablets
B. 45 tablets

4. Ordinary units of weight and volume are used to describe the quantity of most drugs. Specialized units are applied to certain drugs derived from natural sources. These drugs are frequently very complex chemically; sometimes they are mixtures of components of varying potency. Their activity is expressed in comparison to a USP reference standard. These USP *units* of activity usually correspond to recognized international units or to units of activity set by the Food and Drug Administration for antibiotics and biological products. While such units are a measure of potency rather than quantity, the relationship between potency and weight of certain drugs has been established. For example, it has been found that each microgram of penicillin V is equivalent to 1.6 potency units.

How many units are equivalent to 250 mg of penicillin V?

_____

400,000 units. Did you recognize that this was a problem in conversion?

Solution:

1 µg = 1.6 units

250 mg × 10^3 µg/mg × 1.6 units/µg = 400,000 units

---

5. A milligram of d-α-tocopherol is equivalent to 1.49 IU of vitamin E. A formula for vitamin E calls for 20 IU per capsule. How many grams of d-α-tocopherol are required in order to make 20 capsules?

- -

0.268 g

Solution:

20 IU/caps × 20 caps = 400 IU (total needed)

$$400 \text{ IU} \times \frac{1 \text{ mg}}{1.49 \text{ IU}} \times \frac{1 \text{ g}}{1000 \text{ mg}} = 0.268 \text{ g}$$

---

6. For the problems that follow, you will need to know that 1 mg of penicillin V = 1600 units.

A. How many kilograms of penicillin V should be used to prepare 55,000 capsules if each one contains 400,000 units of penicillin V?

B. How many milligrams of penicillin V are there in 5 mL of a suspension that contains 80,000 units/mL?

C. A vial of penicillin V contains 200,000 units of penicillin V per milliliter. How many milliliters will contain 1.5 g of penicillin V?

D. How many grams of penicillin V should be used to prepare 12.5 mL of a suspension containing 200,000 units of penicillin V per milliliter?

_____

A. 13.75 kg
B. 250 mg
C. 12.0 mL
D. 1.56 g

7. Density is defined as the mass per unit-volume of a particular substance:

$$\text{density} = \frac{\text{mass}}{\text{volume}}$$

The units of density depend, of course, on the units used to denote mass and volume. In the metric system, density is usually expressed in terms of grams per milliliter.

Since volume is a function of temperature, density is too. However, for purposes of calculation for prescription compounding, we ignore these temperature effects, since the error so introduced is small and does not materially increase the error of our final result. Thus, while the density of water at 25°C is actually 0.997 g/mL, we use a value of 1.00 g/mL in our calculations.

8. Certain pharmaceutical formulas list all the ingredients by weight, despite the fact that some may be liquids and are therefore more conveniently measured by volume. For example, a formula calls for 2.75 g of methyl salicylate, a liquid. In order to convert this weight to a volume, we need a statement of equivalence. This is provided by the density. The density of methyl

salicylate is 1.18 g/mL. In other words, 1 mL of methyl salicylate weighs 1.18 g, or

1.18 g methyl salicylate = 1 mL methyl salicylate

To convert 2.75 g of methyl salicylate to a volume:

$$2.75 \text{ g} \times \frac{1 \text{ mL}}{1.18 \text{ g}} = 2.33 \text{ mL}$$

Just in case this operation looks like sleight of hand, let us take another look at the fraction 1 mL/1.18 g. If I had 1 mL of methyl salicylate in one vial and 1.18 g of methyl salicylate in another, the amounts in both vials would be identical since 1.18 g is the weight of 1 mL. Thus "1 mL" and "1.18 g" are merely different ways of describing the same quantity of methyl salicylate. The fraction 1 mL/1.18 g is therefore equal to unity, and multiplying by this fraction converts weight to volume.

The density of chloroform is 1.48 g/mL, and that of ether is 0.715 g/mL. For each of these liquids, write an equation that relates weight and volume.

– –

Chloroform: 1.48 g = 1 mL
Ether: 0.715 g = 1 mL

9. A prescription for 60 g of an ointment contains 3 g of light mineral oil. The density of light mineral oil is 0.850 g/mL. The density of the finished ointment is 0.975 g/mL. Which of the following expressions will allow us to determine the volume of light mineral oil that should be used for this prescription? Why are the others incorrect?

A. $3.00 \text{ g} \times \dfrac{1 \text{ mL}}{0.850 \text{ g}} =$

B. $3.00 \text{ g} \times \dfrac{0.850 \text{ g}}{1 \text{ mL}} =$

C. $60.0 \text{ g} \times \dfrac{1 \text{ mL}}{0.850 \text{ g}} =$

D. $3.00 \text{ g} \times \dfrac{1 \text{ mL}}{0.975 \text{ g}} =$

A. Correct because 3.00 g is the amount of light mineral oil we must work with; the fraction 1 mL/0.850 g is equal to unity and the result will be expressed in milliliters.
B. Incorrect because the fraction, although equal to unity, is inverted, so that the result will be expressed as g^2/mL, not milliliters.
C. Incorrect because we do not have 60.0 g of light mineral oil, only 3.00 g.
D. Incorrect because of the fraction 1 mL/0.975 g. 0.975 g/mL is the density of the ointment not of light mineral oil. One mL of light mineral oil does not weigh 0.975 g, so that the fraction is not equal to unity. Consequently, this formula leads not only to an alteration of units but an alteration of quantity as well.

10. If 25.0 g of olive oil are required for a prescription, what volume should be used? (Density of olive oil = 0.910 g/mL.)

27.5 mL

Solution:

$$25.0 \text{ g} \times \dfrac{1 \text{ mL}}{0.910 \text{ g}} = 27.5 \text{ mL}$$

11. How many grams would 2 fluidounces of peanut oil (density = 0.917 g/mL) weigh?

54.3 g

Solution:

2 fluidounces = 59.2 mL

59.2 mL × 0.917 g/mL = 54.3 g

---

12. From these examples it is evident that conversion from weight to volume, or from volume to weight, can be accomplished using the density of the material under consideration. Most often, however, reference sources will not list density; specific gravity will be given instead. Specific gravity (sp g) may be defined as the ratio of the density of a substance to that of some reference material. Water is used as the reference for liquids and solids:

$$\text{sp g} = \frac{\text{density of substance}}{\text{density of water}}$$

Both densities should be expressed in the same units, so that specific gravity is a dimensionless quantity. It should be noted that the specific gravity, as such, cannot be used in converting between weight and volume. We can work only with density and the units must be explicitly stated. However, we may use the definition of specific gravity to find density which can then be employed in conversion calculations.

The specific gravity of glycerin is 1.25. Let us calculate its density in the metric system:

$$\text{sp g} = \frac{\text{density of glycerin}}{\text{density of water}}$$

density of glycerin = sp g × density of water

= 1.25 × 1.00 g/mL = 1.25 g/mL

The density, in g/mL, is numerically equal to the specific gravity. This is not true for other units. For example, the density of glycerin in the apothecary system is 569 grains per fluidounce. Only when density is expressed as g/mL are density and specific gravity numerically equal.

The specific gravity of acetone is 0.788. The density of this material is

A.   0.788 gr/fluidounce
B.   0.788 gr/minim
C.   0.788 g/L
D.   0.788 g/mL

D is correct. Specific gravity is equal to density expressed as g/mL.

---

13. The specific gravity of white petrolatum is 0.850. What weight of this substance will fill an ointment jar whose capacity is 1/2 ounce? (*Hint*: Use the approximate equivalent 1 fluidounce = 30 mL for calculations involving container capacities. In this case, 1/2 ounce = 15 mL.)

12.8 g

Solution:

With a sp g of 0.850, the density is 0.850 g/mL.

$$15.0 \text{ mL} \times 0.850 \text{ g/mL} = 12.8 \text{ g}$$

---

14. A formula calls for 0.623 kg of an oil whose specific gravity is 0.900. How many milliliters should be used?

----

692 mL

Solution:

$$623 \text{ g} \times \frac{1 \text{ mL}}{0.900 \text{ g}} = 692 \text{ mL}$$

---

15. A prescription contains 88.8 mL of hydrochloric acid (sp g = 1.18), which costs $2.20 per pound. What is the cost of the quantity used in the prescription?

$0.51

Solution:

$$88.8 \text{ mL} \times 1.18 \text{ g/mL} = 105 \text{ g hydrochloric acid}$$

$$\frac{454 \text{ g}}{\$2.20} = \frac{105 \text{ g}}{j}$$

$$j = \$0.51$$

---

16. If you want more practice, try these:

A. The specific gravity of an oil is 0.930. How much will 12.0 mL weigh?

B. If the specific gravity of a liquid is 1.10, how many milliliters would 27.0 kg occupy?

C. A formula calls for 1.32 g of an oil whose specific gravity is 0.886. How many microliters should be used?

A.   11.2 g
B.   24,500 mL

C.   1490 μL

---

17. Do all the problems in this frame before verifying your answers. Be certain to write units down and use them. Estimate your result or perform some other kind of check where possible.

A.   How many 2-mg tablets of a drug contain 3/4 gr of the drug?

B.   A prescription calls for 120 mL of a suspension in water containing 0.75 mg of prednisone per milliliter of finished product. How many 5-mg prednisone tablets should the pharmacist use to provide the drug needed to make this prescription?

C.   A pure vitamin D substance has a potency of 40 million USP units of vitamin D per gram. A batch of cod liver oil was assayed and was found to contain 9.70 μg of pure vitamin D in 5.00 mL. How many USP units of vitamin D were present in each cubic centimeter of the oil?

D.   A hospital pharmacist plans to manufacture a liter of a solution containing 10,000 units of nystatin in each mL of solution. How many grams would be needed? (Assume that each mg is equivalent to 4400 Nystatin Units.)

E. If 1 mg of penicillin V is equivalent to 1600 units, and 240 mL of penicillin V suspension contains 12.0 g of penicillin V, how many units will 2.5 mL contain?

F. If an eye ointment is to contain the potency of 500 units of bacitracin (an antibiotic) per gram, how many grams of bacitracin should be used to prepare 500 g of the ointment? Assume that each mg of the antibiotic are equivalent to 40 Bacitracin Units (BU).

G. A prescription calls for 10.0 g of citric acid syrup, a liquid whose specific gravity is 1.17. What volume of citric acid syrup should be used?

H. The specific gravity of an oil is 0.812. How many cubic centimeters should be used to fill a prescription that calls for 9 g?

I. A formula calls for 3.22 kg of an oil whose specific gravity is 0.922. How many milliliters should be used?

J. A formula calls for 0.752 L of an oil whose specific gravity is 0.950. How many kilograms will the oil weigh?

K. Carbon tetrachloride costs \$3.00 for a 1-lb bottle. What is the cost of 3 fluidounces? (The specific gravity of carbon tetrachloride is 1.59.)

- -

A. 24 tablets
B. 18 tablets
C. 77.6 units/cc
D. 2.27 g
E. 200,000 units
F. 6.25 g
G. 8.55 mL
H. 11.1 cc
I. 3490 mL
J. 0.714 kg
K. \$0.93

Solutions:

A. $3/4 \text{ gr} \times 64.8 \text{ mg/gr} \times \dfrac{1 \text{ tablet}}{2 \text{ mg}} = 24$ tablets

B. $120 \text{ mL} \times 0.75 \text{ mg/mL} = 90$ mg

$90 \text{ mg} \times \dfrac{1 \text{ tablet}}{5 \text{ mg}} = 18$ tablets

C. $1 \text{ g} = 40 \times 10^6$ units

$9.70 \text{ μg} \times \dfrac{1 \text{ g}}{10^6 \text{ μg}} \times (40 \times 10^6) \text{ units/g} = 388$ units in 5 mL

$\dfrac{388 \text{ units}}{5 \text{ mL}} = 77.6$ units/mL

D. $10{,}000 \text{ NU/mL} \times 1000 \text{ mL} \times \dfrac{1 \text{ mg}}{4400 \text{ NU}} \times \dfrac{1 \text{ g}}{1000 \text{ mg}} = 2.27$ g

E. $\dfrac{12.0\ \text{g}}{240\ \text{mL}} = \dfrac{j}{2.5\ \text{mL}}$

   $j = 0.125\ \text{g} = 125\ \text{mg present in 5 mL}$

   $125\ \text{mg} \times 1600\ \text{units/mg} = 200{,}000\ \text{units}$

F. $500\ \text{BU/g} \times 500\ \text{g} \times \dfrac{1\ \text{mg}}{40\ \text{BU}} \times \dfrac{1\ \text{g}}{1000\ \text{mg}} = 6.25\ \text{g}$

G. $10.0\ \text{g} \times \dfrac{1\ \text{mL}}{1.17\ \text{g}} = 8.55\ \text{mL}$

H. $9\ \text{g} \times \dfrac{1\ \text{mL}}{0.812\ \text{g}} = 11.1\ \text{cc}$

I. $3.22\ \text{kg} \times \dfrac{1000\ \text{g}}{1\ \text{kg}} \times \dfrac{1\ \text{mL}}{0.922\ \text{g}} = 3490\ \text{mL}$

J. $752\ \text{mL} \times \dfrac{0.950\ \text{g}}{1\ \text{mL}} \times \dfrac{1\ \text{kg}}{1000\ \text{g}} = 0.714\ \text{kg}$

K. $3\ \text{f}\text{℥} \times 29.6\ \text{mL/f}\text{℥} \times 1.59\ \text{g/mL} = 141\ \text{g}$

   $\dfrac{\$3.00}{454\ \text{g}} = \dfrac{j}{141\ \text{g}}$

   $j = \$0.93$

CHAPTER FOUR

FORMULAS: THE PRESCRIPTION

In this chapter, we will work with formulas of various kinds. A number of formulas appear in the <u>USP</u> and *National Formulary* (<u>NF</u>) to provide standardization; the composition of products listed in these references should be uniform. These formulas are written for a fixed amount, and if larger or smaller quantities are desired, the formulas have to be scaled accordingly. You will also learn the conventional ways in which prescriptions are written and many of the abbreviations commonly used in prescription writing. Depending on how a prescription formula is represented, simple calculations allow us to determine the quantity of each component to be included.

Learning objectives: after completing this chapter the student should be able to

1. Enlarge and reduce <u>USP</u> formulas.
2. Rewrite a parts formula in terms of quantities to be measured.
3. State the meaning of common abbreviations used in prescription writing.
4. Calculate the quantities needed for a prescription written in terms of a single dosage unit.
5. Calculate the quantities needed for a prescription written in terms of the total quantity desired.

1. Drugs can usually not be taken in pure form. Many of them are so potent that proper measurement of the small doses required would be extremely difficult. A drug product, often called a *drug*

delivery system or *dosage form*, is a mini-system that makes drug administration accurate, convenient and practical. You are probably already somewhat familiar with many types of drug delivery systems.

An example of a *bulk powder* is baby powder, which is applied to the skin directly from the container. Bulk powders are usually not administered internally because it is very difficult for the patient to measure the dose accurately. The problem of controlling the dose is solved by putting a powdered drug or drug mixture into a dosage form that allows the patient to take a premeasured quantity of the product. Capsules, tablets, and divided powders are examples.

A *capsule* is a shell, usually made of gelatin, that contains the active ingredients. When a capsule is swallowed, the gelatin dissolves in the acid environment of the stomach, releasing the powdered material inside. Because each capsule contains a definite, accurately measured quantity of drug, proper dosage is determined by administering the correct number of capsules. Capsules can be prepared by the pharmacist for a prescription. Many commercial capsule products are also manufactured by pharmaceutical companies.

Several types of *tablets* can be prepared. The type most frequently encountered is the *compressed tablet*, which can be manufactured only on an industrial scale. Tablets are designed to break up into fragments when they enter the stomach fluid, allowing the drug to come into contact with the liquid environment. Many people use the word "pill" to describe a tablet. A pill is actually different. It is an older type of preparation, not commonly used anymore, with a round shape.

In the case of a *divided powder*, the drug or drug mixture is wrapped in a folded paper. The patient unfolds the paper and transfers the powder onto a tablespoon where it is mixed with a small amount of water. The concoction is then swallowed and followed with water or some other liquid to wash the powder down. Many drugs have bitter or otherwise unpleasant taste, and divided powders are not as popular as tablets or capsules, which are usually easier and more pleasant to take.

A *solution* contains dissolved drug; solutions taken by mouth are usually administered by teaspoon or tablespoon. A *syrup* is a solution that is sweet and highly viscous. An *elixir* is a pleasant-tasting solution containing water and alcohol. *Spirits* are solutions in alcohol. *Tinctures* are also basically alcoholic solutions, although other solvents may also be present.

Ointments and *pastes* are semisolid preparations intended for application to a body surface like the skin. Pastes contain a high proportion of powdered material. Ointments and pastes are packaged in tubes or jars. *Suppositories* are firm semisolid units that are designed to be inserted into a particular body opening.

Rectal and vaginal suppositories are the most common. After insertion, the suppository either melts or dissolves, and the drug comes in contact with the local fluids and membrane surfaces. Cocoa butter is a natural material frequently used as a base for suppositories prepared extemporaneously by the pharmacist.

These descriptions of dosage forms have been quite brief. They are intended to acquaint you, in a general way, with some characteristics of drug products that may appear in some of our examples. As you work through the rest of the book, refer to this frame to refresh your memory of these dosage forms, if necessary.

2. Formulas for pharmaceutical products list their contents in various ways. A formula for aspirin tablets, for example, may contain the ingredients and quantities for a single tablet. If 500,000 tablets are to be manufactured, the quantities must be scaled up or enlarged. On the other hand, the formula may be written in terms of 500,000 tablets if this is the size of the usual batch. A change in batch size necessitates enlargement or reduction of the formula. This adjustment of formula quantities is made so that each tablet has the desired composition, regardless of the number of tablets produced in that batch. Of course, the same considerations apply to other dosage forms, such as capsules and suppositories. These dosage forms are alike in that a particular number of units (such as 2 tablets, 1 suppository, etc.) are administered in order to supply a dose. They are called *unit dosage forms*.

Formulas for *bulk dosage forms*, such as ointments and solutions, generally list components in quantities that will yield a definite final weight or volume. Those in the USP are for 1000 g or mL. If some other quantity is desired, the formula must be reduced or enlarged. This adjustment is made so that each gram or milliliter of the finished product has the desired composition, regardless of the size of the batch.

A. When the formula for a unit dosage form (such as a tablet) is reduced or enlarged, both the original and new formula, must have the same _____ per _____ .

B. When the formula for a bulk dosage form (such as a solution) is reduced or enlarged, both the original and new formula, must have the same _____ per _____ .

- -

A. composition, unit
B. composition, unit of weight or volume

3. A hospital uses the following formula for prednisolone capsules,
    2.5 mg:

> Prednisolone: 2.5 mg
> Lactose: 0.9 g

This is the formula for one capsule. We wish to rewrite the
formula to yield 1500 capsules.

Before going ahead with this problem, stop and look again at
the formula. The amount of lactose is 0.9 g. As written, this
quantity has one significant figure. Does this mean that the result
of a calculation based on this formula must necessarily have only
one significant figure, too? The answer is an emphatic <u>no</u>! The
rules dealing with significant figures that we covered in Chapter
1 apply to experimental quantities. In other words, they apply to
measurements that have been completed. Listing a quantity in a
formula in a particular way does not limit the accuracy of any
subsequent calculation or any measurement based on the
calculation. The standards for accuracy depend on the nature of
the product and the manipulative procedure to be used, not on the
number of figures in the formula.

In essence, we can consider the formula quantities to be exact
and carry calculations to the number of significant figures
necessary for the particular application. When performing
calculations for prescription work, the result should generally
have three significant figures. Calculations that apply to
large-scale manufacturing must be carried to at least four
significant figures.

A. With prescription calculations, the result should be accurate to
    _____ significant figures.
B. Results of calculations for large-scale manufacturing should be
    accurate to _____ significant figures.

    _____

    A. three
    B. four or more

---

4. Returning to our problem:
    A hospital uses the following formula for prednisolone
    capsules, 2.5 mg:

> Prednisolone: 2.5 mg
> Lactose: 0.9 g

This is the formula for one capsule. How many grams of each
component should be used to make 1500 capsules?

Formulas are most conveniently reduced or enlarged by multiplying the amount of each ingredient by a suitable factor, f.

$$f = \frac{\text{yield of new formula}}{\text{yield of original formula}}$$

The yields must be given in the same units. The factor is dimensionless. In this problem,

$$f = \frac{1500 \text{ capsules}}{1 \text{ capsule}} = 1500$$

For the prednisolone,

2.5 mg $\times$ 1500 = 3750 mg = 3.75 g

Calculate the amount of lactose. Check your result by adding the amounts of prednisolone and lactose and comparing the sum with that of the total weight on one capsule (from the formula) multiplied by 1500.

––––––––––––––––––––––––––––

Lactose: 0.9 g $\times$ 1500 = 1350 g

To check:

Sum of weights:
$$\begin{array}{r} 3.75 \quad \text{g} \\ 1350. \quad\quad \text{g} \\ \hline 1353.75 \quad \text{g} \end{array}$$

Weight of 1500 capsules:

each capsule = 2.5 mg + 900 mg = 902.5 mg

902.5 mg $\times$ 1500 = 1,353,750 mg = 1353.75 g

5. Here is the formula for ergotamine tartrate and caffeine suppositories:

Ergotamine tartrate: 2 mg
Caffeine: 100 mg
Cocoa butter: 1.898 g

This formula is for one suppository. Your firm wishes to manufacture 5000 suppositories. How many grams of each ingredient should be used?

_____

Ergotamine tartrate: 10.00 g
Caffeine: 500.0 g
Cocoa butter: 9490 g

In essence, this type of calculation leads to a revised formula. By stating that the required amount of ergotamine tartrate is 10.00 g, I am emphasizing that the calculation was accurate to four figures. It would also be correct to write "10 g" for the amount of ergotamine tartrate since it is understood that the accuracy of measurement is not limited by the number of figures used in the revised formula.

Solution:

$$f = \frac{5000 \text{ suppositories}}{1 \text{ suppository}} = 5000$$

Ergotamine tartrate: 2 mg $\times$ 5000 = 10,000 mg = 10 g
Caffeine: 0.1 g $\times$ 5000 = 500 g
Cocoa butter: 1.898 g $\times$ 5000 = 9490 g

We can check our calculations by comparing the sum of the weights of the ingredients with the calculated theoretical weight of 5000 suppositories:

Theoretical weight: 2.000 g $\times$ 5000 = 10,000 g

Sum of ingredients:

	10 g
	500 g
	9,490 g
	10,000 g

6. A pharmaceutical manufacturer utilizes the following formula to make 100 capsules:

    Ephedrine sulfate: 30 g
    Amaranth: 1 g
    Lactose: 250 g

    We wish to rewrite the formula (in kilograms) so as to yield 200,000 capsules. Calculate the value of the factor, f.

    _

    $$f = \frac{2 \times 10^5 \text{ caps}}{100 \text{ caps}} = 2000$$

---

7. Now calculate the amounts (in kilograms) in the formula for 200,000 capsules.

    _

    Ephedrine sulfate: 60 kg
    Amaranth: 2 kg
    Lactose: 500 kg

    Solution:

    Ephedrine sulfate: 30 g $\times$ 2000 = 60,000 g = 60 kg
    Amaranth: 1 g $\times$ 2000 = 2000 g = 2 kg
    Lactose: 0.25 kg $\times$ 2000 = 500 kg

    To check:

Sum of weights:	60 kg
	2 kg
	500 kg
	562 kg

Weight of 200,000 caps:

total wt of 100 caps = 281 g

0.281 kg × 2000 = 562 kg

The formula for cherry syrup is

Cherry juice: 475 mL
Sucrose: 800 g
Alcohol: 20 mL
Purified water: a sufficient quantity to make 1000 mL

A pharmacist wishes to prepare 120 mL of this syrup for a prescription. What value of f should be used in reducing the formula?

_____

$$f = \frac{\text{yield of reduced formula}}{\text{yield of original formula}} = \frac{120 \text{ mL}}{1000 \text{ mL}} = 0.12$$

8. What quantity of each ingredient should be used to prepare 120 mL of the syrup?

_____

Cherry juice: 57 mL
Sucrose: 96 g
Alcohol: 2.4 mL
Purified water: a sufficient quantity to make 120 mL

Solution:

Cherry juice: 475 mL × 0.12 = 57 mL
Sucrose: 800 g × 0.12 = 96 g

Alcohol: 20 mL × 0.12 = 2.4 mL

Notice that the exact quantity of water cannot be calculated, since we do not know the volume occupied by the solids in solution. The best we can do is to say "a sufficient quantity to make 120 mL." It is generally true that liquid preparations are completed by adding sufficient diluent to reach the desired volume using an appropriate measuring device. On the other hand, the weight of each ingredient is known and should be indicated in formulas written on a weight basis.

9. The formula for Ringer's solution follows:

Sodium chloride: 8.60 g
Potassium chloride: 0.30 g
Calcium chloride: 0.33 g
Water for injection: a sufficient quantity to make 1000 mL

How much of each ingredient is necessary to make 90 mL of Ringer's solution?

_____

Sodium chloride: 0.774 g
Potassium chloride: 0.0270 g
Calcium chloride: 0.0297 g
Water for injection: a sufficient quantity to make 90.0 mL

Solution:

$$f = \frac{90.0 \text{ mL}}{1000 \text{ mL}} = 0.09$$

Sodium chloride: 8.60 g × 0.09 = 0.774 g
Potassium chloride: 0.30 g × 0.09 = 0.0270 g
Calcium chloride: 0.33 g × 0.09 = 0.0297 g
Water for injection: a sufficient quantity to make 90.0 mL

10. Not all formulas indicate what the final yield will be. For example, the formula for an aromatic concentrate is

Camphor   20 g
Anise oil   5 mL
Alcohol   130 mL

If we desire to make 25.0 mL of this concentrate, we cannot arrive at precise quantities, because the final volume is not given by the formula. It is reasonable in such a case to make a little more than is required and discard the excess. Hopefully, this procedure will not be too expensive.

In this particular case, we can be certain of getting at least 25 mL of concentrate if we use 25 mL of alcohol. What quantities of the other ingredients should be used?

_____

Camphor: 3.84 g
Anise oil: 0.96 mL

Solution:

This problem may be solved by proportion, or by recognizing that reduction of the formula is accomplished by multiplying all quantities by the same dimensionless factor. Since 25 mL of alcohol will be used while the original formula is for 130 mL of alcohol,

$$f = \frac{25 \text{ mL}}{130 \text{ mL}} = 0.192$$

Camphor: 20 g × 0.192 = 3.84 g
Anise oil: 5 mL × 0.192 = 0.96 mL

---

11. The formula for bemegride injection is

Bemegride: 0.5 g
Sodium chloride: 0.9 g
Water for injections: sufficient to produce 100 mL

Your firm wishes to make some of this injection. You have on hand 53 g of bemegride, 0.75 kg of sodium chloride, and unlimited water for injections. How many liters of bemegride injection can you manufacture?

10.6 L

Solution:

Whatever quantity is made, each ingredient will be present in the same ratio to that quantity as in the formula. The quantity made is limited by the ingredient in shortest supply. Water for injections cannot be the limiting ingredient.

The amount of injection that can be made from 53 g of bemegride may be found as follows:

$$\frac{0.5 \text{ g bemegride}}{100 \text{ mL injection}} = \frac{53 \text{ g bemegride}}{j}$$

$j = 10,600$ mL injection

The amount of injection that can be made from 0.75 kg of sodium chloride is

$$\frac{0.9 \text{ g NaCl}}{100 \text{ mL injection}} = \frac{750 \text{ g NaCl}}{j}$$

$j = 83,300$ mL injection

It is apparent that bemegride is the limiting ingredient. Thus 10,600 mL or 10.6 L of the injection can be manufactured.

---

12. In this frame you will be given a formula to make 1000 mL of ferrous sulfate syrup. You will then be asked to calculate the quantities necessary to make 8 fluidounces of the syrup. Before going ahead with the calculation, stop and consider the use to which it will be put. There is no reason whatever to convert all quantities into apothecary units. Such a conversion unnecessarily complicates a simple calculation and introduces more opportunity for arithmetic error. The way to proceed is to use the approximate equivalent for the total volume required; since 1 fluidounce is approximately equivalent to 30 mL, 8 fluidounces $\approx$ 240 mL.

It is not necessary to use a more exact conversion procedure (which would result in a value of 237 mL) for two reasons: (1) Metric graduates have no 237-mL mark.

(2) The more important consideration is that the composition of each milliliter of the syrup be the same as that in the original formula. Use of 240 mL for 8 f℥ does not contradict our requirements for accuracy in prescription compounding, since the ratio of all components in the formula to the finished quantity will not be altered.

From the following formula calculate the quantities required to make 8 f℥ of ferrous sulfate syrup:

Ferrous sulfate: 40 g
Citric acid, hydrous: 2.1 g
Peppermint spirit: 2 mL
Sucrose: 825 g
Purified water: a sufficient quantity to make 1000 mL

––––––––––––––––––––––

Ferrous sulfate: 9.60 g
Citric acid, hydrous: 0.504 g
Peppermint spirit: 0.480 mL
Sucrose: 198 g
Purified water: sufficient to make 240 mL

Solution:

$$f = \frac{240 \text{ mL}}{1000 \text{ mL}} = 0.24$$

Ferrous sulfate: 40 g × 0.24 = 9.60 g
Citric acid hydrous: 2.1 g × 0.24 = 0.504 g
Peppermint spirit: 2 mL × 0.24 = 0.480 mL
Sucrose: 825 g × 0.24 = 198 g
Purified water: sufficient to make 240 mL

13. The formula for iodine tincture USP is

Iodine: 20 g
NaI: 24 g
Alcohol: 500 mL
Purified water: a sufficient quantity to make 1000 mL

What quantity of each ingredient should be used to make one-half fluidounce of iodine tincture?

Iodine: 0.3 g
NaI: 0.36 g
Alcohol: 7.5 mL
Purified water: a sufficient quantity to make 15 mL

Solution:

$$f = \frac{15 \text{ mL}}{1000 \text{ mL}} = 0.015$$

Iodine: 20 g × 0.015 = 0.3 g
NaI: 24 g × 0.015 = 0.36 g
Alcohol: 500 mL × 0.015 = 7.5 mL

14. The formula for sodium phosphate solution is

Sodium phosphate: 755 g
Citric acid: 130 g
Glycerin: 150 mL
Purified water: a sufficient quantity to make 1000 mL

How much of each ingredient should be used to make 90.0 mL of sodium phosphate solution for a prescription?

Sodium phosphate: 68.0 g
Citric acid: 11.7 g
Glycerin: 13.5 mL
Purified water: a sufficient quantity to make 90.0 mL

15. Some formulas are given in terms of *parts* rather than specific units of weight or volume. Such formulas indicate the ratio of ingredient quantities to each other. In a formula given in terms of parts by weight, any unit of weight may be used, but it must be applied to all of the components. In a formula given in parts by volume, any unit of volume may be used, provided that all components have the same units.

Here is the formula for zinc oxide paste written by parts:

Zinc oxide: 1 part
Starch: 1 part
White petrolatum: 2 parts

This formula could be written

Zinc oxide: 1 lb
Starch: 1 lb
White petrolatum: 2 lb

or

Zinc oxide: 1 kg
Starch: 1 kg
White petrolatum: 2 kg

The actual units applied are determined by the units describing the desired quantity.

How much of each ingredient is required to make 60 g of zinc oxide paste?

_ _

Zinc oxide: 15 g
Starch: 15 g
White petrolatum: 30 g

Solution:

To use the formula, we simply replace "parts" by "grams," since our target quantity is 60 g.

Zinc oxide: 1 g
Starch: 1 g
White petrolatum: 2 g
                      ‾‾‾
                       4 g

$$f = \frac{60 \text{ g}}{4 \text{ g}} = 15$$

Zinc oxide: 1 g × 15 = 15 g
Starch: 1 g × 15 = 15 g
White petrolatum: 2 g × 15 = 30 g

The sum of all ingredients is 60 g, the desired quantity.

16. A foot powder has this formula:

Talc: 15 parts
Benzoic acid: 1 part
Bentonite: 3 parts

Rewrite the formula so that it will yield 25 kg of foot powder. (Your results should contain four significant figures.)

————————————————————

Talc: 19.74 kg
Benzoic acid: 1.316 kg
Bentonite: 3.948 kg

Solution:

The parts formula may be rewritten

Talc: 15 kg
Benzoic acid: 1 kg
Bentonite: 3 kg

This makes a total of 19 kg.

$$f = \frac{25}{19} = 1.316$$

Talc: 15 kg × 1.316 =   19.74 kg
Benzoic acid: 1 kg × 1.316 =   1.316 kg
Bentonite: 3 kg × 1.316 =   3.948 kg
                                  25.00 kg

17. The formula for an analgesic powder is:

> Aspirin: 6 parts
> Phenacetin: 3 parts
> Caffeine: 1 part

All quantities are based on weight. How many grams of aspirin should be used to prepare 1.25 kg of the powder?

750 g

Solution:

$$f = \frac{1250 \text{ g}}{10 \text{ g}} = 125$$

6 g × 125 = 750 g

18. The formula for yellow ointment may be written

> Yellow wax: 1 part
> Petrolatum: 19 parts

How many kilograms of yellow ointment can be prepared from 660 g of yellow wax?

13.2 kg

Solution:

$$\frac{1}{20} = \frac{0.660 \text{ kg}}{j}$$

$j = 13.2$ kg

19. A prescription is a legal request for medication, which may be written by a properly licensed physician, dentist, podiatrist, or veterinarian. It is helpful to explore the form and content of the prescription, since many of our calculations will be concerned with prescription compounding.

   On the prescription will be found the date, the name and address of the patient, the drugs to be used and type of preparation, directions to the patient, refill information, and the signature, address, and (for controlled drugs) BNDD registry number of the prescriber.

   We will not explore the legal issues involved in handling the prescription. Our discussion will be limited to those aspects relating to calculations.

20. A fairly uniform format, shown in Table 4–1, is used by prescribers to indicate the active ingredient(s), quantity to be dispensed, the form of medication (in other words, the prescription formula), instructions to the pharmacist, and the directions for use by the patient. The directions to the patient relate to the dosage of the prescribed drug(s) and are considered in detail in the Chapter 5.

Table 4–1. Standard Prescription Format

Typical Prescription	Information
℞	The prescription symbol
Aspirin 7.2 g Phenacetin 5.0 g	Names and quantities of prescribed drugs
Mix. Divide into 12 capsules	Instructions to the pharmacist
Sig: caps I t.i.d. p.c.	Directions to the patient (also known as the signa)

After reviewing the table, fill in the blanks. The major parts of the prescription are

    1. The symbol, _____ .
    2. Names and quantities of d_____ .
    3. Instructions to the p_____ .
    4. Directions to the p_____ .

———————————————————

1. ℞
2. drugs
3. pharmacist
4. patient

21. As you can see from the example in the frame 20, certain abbreviations are used routinely in writing prescriptions. They are usually derived from Latin phrases. The type of preparation to be compounded or dispensed (commonly called the dosage form) is one of the things indicated in the directions to the pharmacist. Table 4–2 lists many of the abbreviations, some of which are derived from the Latin, and their meaning.

Table 4–2. Dosage Form Abbreviations

Abbreviation or Term	Meaning
caps	capsule
chart	divided powder; powder in a paper
elix	elixir
pulv, pulvis	powder, bulk powder
sol	solution
supp	suppository
susp	suspension
syr	syrup
tab	tablet
ung, unguentum	ointment

Sometimes these abbreviations are followed by periods and sometimes they are not. Either upper case or lower case letters may be used. These generalizations are true for all of the terms and abbreviations used in prescription writing.

Also included in the directions to the pharmacist are terms such as those listed in Table 4–3. Go through the table and learn their meaning.

Table 4–3. Abbreviations Used in Directions to the Pharmacist

Term or Abbreviation	Meaning
disp	dispense
f, ft	make
M	mix
No., #	number of units to be prepared or dispensed
S.A., secundum artem	according to art (a vague phrase meaning roughly "use your skill and judgment")

Translate the following phrases into good English:

A. ft. ung.
B. disp tab #24
C. M. f. sol.
D. ft chart No. xxxvi SA

– –

A. Make an ointment.
B. Dispense 24 tablets.
C. Mix and make a solution.
D. Make 36 divided powders according to art.

22. Certain abbreviations appearing in the prescription formula are listed in Table 4–4. The periods that follow the abbreviations shown in the table may be omitted in prescription writing.

Table 4–4. Abbreviations in the Prescription Formula

Latin Abbreviation	Meaning
a̅a̅	of each
aq., aqua	water
aq. dest.	distilled water
aq. pur.	purified water
q.s.	a sufficient quantity
q.s. ad	a sufficient quantity to make
a̅a̅ qs ad	a sufficient quantity of each to make

The first item in the table, "$\overline{aa}$," is used when two or more ingredients are present in the same amount. They are listed sequentially with the symbol placed next to the last item of the group to which it refers.

"$\overline{aa}$ qs ad" tells you to add more than one substance to achieve a specified total weight or volume. It is assumed that these substances will contribute equally. In other words, the missing weight or volume is divided equally between the ingredients identified.

Rewrite the following prescription omitting all abbreviations, so that it makes sense. How much petrolatum should be weighed?

R

Starch	
Talc $\overline{aa}$	5.0 g
Lanolin	10.0 g
Petrolatum qs ad	60.0 g

Ft. ung.

———————————————————

R

Starch	5.0 g	
Talc	5.0 g	(5.0 g "of each" of starch and talc)
Lanolin	10.0 g	
Petrolatum: qs ad	60.0 g.	

Make an ointment.

40.0 g of petrolatum should be weighed.

23. Prescriptions written in the metric system specify quantities using decimal notation. If units are omitted, and the prescription is written in decimal notation, it is understood that metric units are to be employed: solids are weighed in terms of grams, and liquids are measured in milliliters.

R̵
    Zinc oxide
    Talc
    Starch $\overline{aa}$ 5.0
    Lanolin
    Petrolatum $\overline{aa}$ qs ad 60.0

How much petrolatum should be used? (All ingredients are solids.)

————————————————————

22.5 g

Solution:

Since the materials are all solids and the quantities are written using decimal notation, they represent weight in grams. 5.0 g of each of zinc oxide, talc and starch makes a total of 15.0 g. The expression "$\overline{aa}$ qs ad" directs that a sufficient quantity of each be used, or, in other words, that the ingredients under the jurisdiction of this abbreviation should be given an equal share in arriving at the final weight. The remaining 45.0 g are shared equally by the lanolin and petrolatum, so we need 22.5 g of each of these.

---

24. In compounding dosage forms such as capsules and powders in paper, the pharmacist weighs sufficient of each drug to make all of the required doses. The drugs are combined into a homogeneous mix that is then divided equally among the units being prepared.

R̵
    Calcium carbonate
    Sodium bicarbonate $\overline{aa}$ 5.0
    Charcoal   0.4
Div in chart No. x

This prescription contains the formula for 10 powders. The pharmacist is directed to weigh the quantities indicated, combine them, and then divide the mass into 10 papers (the abbreviation "div" means divide). The quantity of a drug that will be contained in each powder paper may be calculated by dividing the total weight of the drug by the number of dosage units.

For example, the amount of calcium carbonate in each powder is

$$\frac{5.00 \text{ g}}{10 \text{ units}} = 0.50 \text{ g/unit (or g/powder paper)}$$

Calculate the total weight of material that will be contained in each powder paper.

1.04 g

Solution:

The total weight of powder in the formula is

Calcium carbonate:	5.0 g
Sodium bicarbonate:	5.0 g
Charcoal:	0.4 g
	10.4 g

$$\frac{10.4 \text{ g}}{10 \text{ powder papers}} = 1.04 \text{ g/powder paper}$$

---

25. Instead of giving the formula for the desired number of dosage units, the prescription may give the formula for a single unit. To calculate the amount of each drug to be measured, it is necessary to multiply the quantity per unit by the number of units.

℞

Aspirin		30
Cocoa butter qs ad	2	

Ft suppositories, d.t.d. #6

The vertical line represents the decimal point. (Some prescription blanks are printed this way.) Both materials are solids, so that the unit of measurement for both is the gram. Thus the amount of aspirin is 300 mg (0.3 g). The abbreviation "d.t.d."

means "give such doses" and indicates the number of units that are to be compounded or dispensed. Whenever "d.t.d." is used, the formula is written for a single unit and must be enlarged by the pharmacist.

Calculate the quantity of each material that should be used to compound the prescription above.

_____

Aspirin: 1.80 g
Cocoa butter: 10.2 g

Solution:

To calculate the total amount of aspirin needed, multiply the content of each unit (suppository) by the number of units:

300 mg × 6 = 1800 mg = 1.80 g

Total wt = 2 g per suppository, of which 300 mg is aspirin. Thus

2.00 g total − 0.30 g aspirin = 1.70 g cocoa butter

1.70 g × 6 = 10.2 g

To check:

Sum of weights: 1.80 g + 10.2 g = 12.0 g

Weight of 6 suppositories: 2 g × 6 = 12 g

26. Calculate the quantity of each drug needed for the prescription that follows. All are solids.

℞
Phenobarbital	0.03
Belladonna extract	0.015
Sodium bicarbonate	0.6

Ft. caps d.t.d. No. XXXVI

Phenobarbital: 1.08 g
Belladonna extract: 0.540 g
Sodium bicarbonate: 21.6 g

Solution:

Phenobarbital: 0.03 g/caps × 36 caps = 1.08 g
Belladonna extract: 0.015 g/caps × 36 caps = 0.540 g
Sodium bicarbonate: 0.6 g/caps × 36 caps = 21.6 g

To check:

Weight of each capsule:
    0.030 g
    0.015 g
    0.600 g
    ―――――
    0.645 g

Weight of 36 caps: 0.645 g/caps × 36 caps = 23.2 g

Sum of weights:
     1.08 g
     0.54 g
    21.6 g
    ――――――
    23.2 g

---

27. Here is a prescription for a liquid preparation in which the formula is written for one unit (the unit in this case is 5 mL, the volume of a teaspoon):

℞

Sodium bromide	0.6 g
Syrup	2.5 mL
Aq dest qs ad	5.0 mL

Ft sol d.t.d. No. 24

Before compounding, the pharmacist must enlarge the formula to find the weights and volumes necessary for 24 such units.
    Perform this calculation.

_____

Sodium bromide: 14.4 g
Syrup: 60.0 mL
Distilled water: sufficient to make 120 mL of solution

Solution:

sodium bromide: 0.6 g × 24 = 14.4 g
syrup: 2.5 mL × 24 = 60.0 mL
total volume: 5.0 mL × 24 = 120 mL

---

28. State how much sodium bicarbonate (a solid) and elixir
phenobarbital (a liquid) should be used to prepare this solution:

℞

Sodium bicarbonate	0.4
Elixir phenobarbital	2.5
Aromatic elixir qs ad	5.0

M Ft sol 180 mL

_____

Sodium bicarbonate: 14.4 g
Elixir phenobarbital: 90.0 mL

Solution:

The formula must be enlarged to yield 180 mL

$$f = \frac{180 \text{ mL}}{5 \text{ mL}} = 36$$

Sodium bicarbonate: 0.4 g × 36 = 14.4 g
Elixir phenobarbital: 2.5 mL × 36 = 90.0 mL

29. Use these problems involving prescription formulas for further practice and review.

A.   ℞

        Sodium phenobarbital   15 mg
        Tincture belladonna   0.5 mL
        Aromatic elixir qs ad   5.0 mL
  d.t.d. No. 48

What quantities should be used to prepare this prescription?

B.   ℞

        Hydrocortisone   0.3 g
        Lactose
  Ft caps Div in caps #40

How many micrograms of hydrocortisone are contained in each capsule?

C.   ℞

        Dilaudid   0.003
        Aspirin   300
  d.t.d. caps No. LXIV

How many tablets, each containing 4 mg of Dilaudid, should be used to supply the Dilaudid for this prescription?

D. ℞

       Cinnamon water   1.5 mL
       Elixir phenobarbital   2.5 mL
       Aromatic elixir qs ad   5.0 mL
Dispense 120 mL

What quantity of each ingredient should be measured?

E. A formula for 12 bismuth subsalicylate suppositories calls for

Bismuth subsalicylate 1.4 g
Cocoa butter qs ad 24 g

How many kilograms of cocoa butter are needed for 150 suppositories?

F. ℞

       Dextroamphetamine sulfate   7.5 mg
       Lactose qs ad   300 mg
d.t.d. caps No. 36

How many tablets, each containing 10 mg of dextroamphetamine sulfate, should be used for this prescription?

_____

A. Sodium phenobarbital: 720 mg
   Tincture belladonna: 24 mL
   Aromatic elixir: qs ad 240 mL

B. 7500 µg
C. 48 tablets
D. Cinnamon water: 36 mL
    Elixir phenobarbital: 60 mL
    Aromatic elixir: qs ad 120 mL
E. 0.2825 kg
F. 27 tablets

30. The questions in this frame review all of the material in this
     chapter. Answer all of them before verifying your results. Check
     your answers where possible. Use estimation to avoid gross errors
     in calculation.

A. R$_X$

    Coal tar ointment
    Disp. 30.0 g

    The pharmacist must prepare the coal tar ointment for this
prescription. What quantity of each ingredient should be used?
The formula for coal tar ointment is

Coal tar: 10 g
Polysorbate 80: 5 g
Zinc oxide paste: a sufficient quantity to make 1000 g

B. The formula for green soap tincture is

    Lavender oil: 20 mL
    Green soap: 650 g
    Alcohol: a sufficient quantity to make 1000 mL

    How much lavender oil and green soap should be used to
prepare 12.5 L of green soap tincture?

C. Here is the formula for placebo tablets:

Lactose: 100 g
Sucrose: 150 g
Starch, direct compressing formula: 250 g
Magnesium sulfate: 0.5 g
        Yield: 1000 tablets

    Rewrite the formula so as to yield 50,000 tablets. Express
quantities in kilograms.

D. The formula for camphorated parachlorophenol is

Parachlorophenol: 7 parts
Camphor: 13 parts

    What quantities should be used to make 150 g of
camphorated parachlorophenol?

E. Compound undecylenic acid ointment contains

Undecylenic acid: 50 g
Zinc undecylenate: 200 g
Polyethylene glycol ointment: 750

    How much compound undecylenic acid ointment could be
made from 2.2 kg of undecylenic acid, 8.5 kg of zinc
undecylenate, and 30 kg of polyethylene glycol ointment?

F. ℞
        Prednisone   2.75 mg
        Acetylsalicylic acid   0.60 g
    Ft caps d.t.d. XXIX

Although you do not have any pure prednisone available, you do have 5-mg tablets. How many tablets would you use in compounding this prescription?

G.   R̽

Sodium salicylate	0.6 g
Sodium bicarbonate	0.15 g
Elixir lactated pepsin qs ad	15 mL

M. d.t.d. No. 8

What quantity of each ingredient should be used for this prescription?

H.   R̽

Zinc oxide	
Starch	
Calamine $\overline{aa}$	12 g
Sodium bicarbonate qs ad	44 g

Ft. pulv

How many grams of sodium bicarbonate should be used to prepare 12 g of this mixture?

I.   R̽

Calcium carbonate	0.5 g
Magnesium trisilicate	0.3 g
Bismuth subcarbonate qs ad	1.2 g

dtd chart #XLII

What quantity of each ingredient should be weighed for this prescription?

J.   ℞

   Calcium gluconate   48 g
   Thiamin   8 g
Div. in caps Ft. No. 60

How many milligrams of thiamin will each capsule contain?

K.   The formula for zinc gelatin is

   Zinc oxide: 100 g
   Gelatin: 150 g
   Glycerin: 400 g
   Purified water: 350 g

How much of each ingredient should be used to make 240 g
of zinc gelatin?

L.   The formula for nitromersol solution is

   Nitromersol: 2 g
   Sodium hydroxide: 0.4 g
   Monohydrated sodium carbonate: 4.25 g
   Purified water: a sufficient quantity to make 1000 mL

What quantities should be used to make 90 mL of
nitromersol solution for a prescription?

M. A formula for a dusting powder contains

> Salicylic acid: 1 part
> Benzoic acid: 3 parts
> Starch: 20 parts

How many grams of each ingredient should be used to make 12 kg of dusting powder?

N. ℞

> Dexamethasone   0.045 g
> Lactose qs

Ft caps. Div in caps No. 68

How many tablets of dexamethasone, each containing 0.75 mg, should be used to provide the drug for this prescription?

O. ℞

> Sodium bromide   1.2 g
> Syrup tolu   2.0 mL
> Syrup wild cherry qs ad 5.0 mL

d.t.d. #24

How many grams of sodium bromide should be used in filling this prescription?

_____

A. Coal tar: 0.300 g
Polysorbate 80: 0.150 g
Zinc oxide paste: 29.6 g
B. Lavender oil: 250 mL

Green soap: 8125 g
C. Lactose: 5 kg
Sucrose: 7.5 kg
Starch : 12.5 kg
Magnesium sulfate: 0.025 kg
D. Parachlorophenol: 52.5 g
Camphor: 97.5 g
E. 40 kg
F. 16 tablets
G. Sodium salicylate: 4.80 g
Sodium bicarbonate: 1.20 g
Elixir lactated pepsin: sufficient quantity to make 120 mL
H. 2.18 g
I. Calcium carbonate: 21.0 g
Magnesium trisilicate: 12.6 g
Bismuth subcarbonate; 16.8 g
J. 133 mg
K. Zinc oxide: 24 g
Gelatin: 36 g
Glycerin: 96 g
Purified water: 84 g
L. Nitromersol: 0.18 g
Sodium hydroxide: 0.036 g
Monohydrated sodium carbonate: 0.383 g
Purified water: sufficient to make 90 mL
M. Salicylic acid: 500 g
Benzoic acid: 1,500 g
Starch: 10,000 g
N. 60 tablets
O. 28.8 g

Solutions:

A. $f = \dfrac{30 \text{ g}}{1000 \text{ g}} = 0.03$

Coal tar: 10 g × 0.03 = 0.300 g
Polysorbate 80: 5 g × 0.03 = 0.150 g
Zinc oxide paste: 985 g × 0.03 = 29.6 g

Total weight = 30.0 g

B. $f = \dfrac{12.5 \text{ L}}{1 \text{ L}} = 12.5$

Lavender oil: 20 ml × 12.5 = 250 ml
Green soap: 650 g × 12.5 = 8125 g

C. $f = \dfrac{50{,}000 \text{ tablets}}{1000 \text{ tablets}} = 50$

Lactose: 0.1 kg × 50 = 5 kg
Sucrose: 0.15 kg × 50 = 7.5 kg
Starch: 0.25 kg × 50 = 12.5 kg
Magnesium sulfate: 0.0005 kg × 50 = 0.025 kg

D. The total number of parts is 20. This may be equated to 20 g:

$$f = \dfrac{150 \text{ g}}{20 \text{ g}} = 7.5$$

Parachlorophenol: 7 g × 7.5 = 52.5 g
Camphor: 13 g × 7.5 = 97.5 g

E. The formula makes 1000 g

Undecylenic acid:

$$\dfrac{50 \text{ g}}{1000 \text{ g}} = \dfrac{2.2 \text{ kg}}{j}$$

j = 44 kg compound undecylenic acid ointment

Zinc undecylenate:

$$\dfrac{200 \text{ g}}{1000 \text{ g}} = \dfrac{8.5 \text{ kg}}{j}$$

j = 42.5 kg compound undecylenic acid ointment

Polyethylene glycol ointment:

$$\dfrac{750 \text{ g}}{1000 \text{ g}} = \dfrac{30 \text{ kg}}{j}$$

j = 40 kg compound undecylenic acid ointment

Only 40 kg of compound undecylenic acid ointment can be made.

F. 2.75 mg/caps × 29 caps × $\dfrac{1 \text{ tablet}}{5 \text{ mg}}$ = 16 tablets

G. Sodium salicylate: 0.6 g × 8 = 4.80 g
Sodium bicarbonate: 0.15 g × 8 = 1.20 g
Total volume: 15.0 mL × 8 = 120 mL

H. Since 12 g of each of the other components are used to make 44 g of the mixture, the amount of sodium bicarbonate is

$$44 \text{ g} - (3)(12) \text{ g} = 8 \text{ g}$$

$$\frac{8 \text{ g}}{44 \text{ g}} = \frac{j}{12 \text{ g}}$$

$$j = 2.18 \text{ g}$$

I. Calcium carbonate: 0.5 g × 42 = 21.0 g
Magnesium trisilicate: 0.3 g × 42 = 12.6 g
Bismuth subcarbonate: 0.4 g × 42 = 16.8 g

J. 8000 mg/60 caps = 133 mg/caps

K. $f = \dfrac{240 \text{ g}}{1000 \text{ g}} = 0.24$

Zinc oxide: 100 g × 0.24 = 24 g

Gelatin: 150 g × 0.24 = 36 g

Glycerin: 400 g × 0.24 = 96 g

Purified water: 350 g × 0.24 = 84 g

L. $f = \dfrac{90 \text{ g}}{1000 \text{ g}} = 0.09$

Nitromersol: 2 g × 0.09 = 0.18 g

Sodium hydroxide: 0.4 g × 0.09 = 0.036 g

Monohydrated sodium carbonate: 4.25 g × 0.09 = .383 g

M. $f = \dfrac{12{,}000 \text{ g}}{24 \text{ g}} = 500$

Salicylic acid: 1 g × 500 = 500 g

Benzoic acid: 3 g × 500 = 1500 g

Starch: 20 g × 500 = 10,000 g

N. $45 \text{ mg} \times \dfrac{1 \text{ tablet}}{0.75 \text{ mg}} = 60 \text{ tablets}$

O. 1.2 g × 24 = 28.8 g

CHAPTER FIVE

DOSAGE

In this chapter we continue our study of the prescription, concentrating on calculations that relate to dosage. You will learn some more abbreviations derived from Latin that are used to indicate directions for use by the patient. The capacities of household measuring devices for taking medication will be reviewed and you will calculate dosages based on body weight and surface area. In general, dosage calculations can be carried to two significant figures and approximate equivalents are used when converting from one measurement system to another.

Learning objectives: after completing this chapter the student should be able to

1. Understand dosing directions written in shorthand using Latin abbreviations.
2. Calculate the number of dosage units or amount of liquid to dispense from the dose and dosing frequency.
3. Determine the dose to be administered from a prescription formula.
4. Calculate the number of drops needed to supply a predetermined liquid dose from the number of drops in a fixed volume.
5. Calculate the flow rate, in drops/minute, for an intravenous infusion from the rate of drug administration.
6. Calculate doses from a knowledge of body weight or surface area.

1. It is the pharmacist's obligation to check the dosage of all drugs dispensed on prescription in order to prevent accidental overdose. The pharmacist must also make certain that the patient understands how the medication is to be taken. The directions to the patient that appear on the prescription label must be written in a way that is clear and unambiguous.

Included in the directions to the patient are:
(1) the number of dosage units in each dose (e.g., 1 capsule, 2 teaspoonfuls, 15 drops);
(2) the frequency with which the medication is to be taken (e.g., three times a day, every four hours);
(3) additional, clarifying instructions (e.g., after meals, with water).

The directions for use by the patient include:

A. _____
B. _____
C. _____

— —

A. Number of dosage units in each dose
B. Frequency of administration
C. Additional clarifying instructions

2. The number of dosage units in each dose is usually specified in Arabic numerals but sometimes roman numerals are used; they may be written in either capital or small letters and follow the name of the dosage form. The final "i" in a Roman numeral is sometimes replaced by a "j".

1 tab (1 tablet)
caps ij (2 capsules)

What is meant by "chart III"?

— —

Three powders in paper.

3. Latin abbreviations are often used to describe the frequency of administration. Some of the commonly used abbreviations are listed in Table 5–1. Sometimes periods are omitted from the abbreviated terms.

Table 5–1. Latin Abbreviations Related to Dosage Frequency

Latin Abbreviation	Meaning
d.	day
h.	hour(s)
q.	every
q. 4 h.	every 4 hours
q.d	every day
b.i.d.	twice a day
t.i.d.	three times a day
q.i.d.	four times a day (here the "q" does not stand for "every")
h.s.	at bedtime
stat	immediately; at once

As an example, let us consider these directions to the patient:

Sig: 1 tab q 3 h [Take one (1) tablet every three (3) hours.]
Sig: Chart I h.s. [Take one (1) powder at bedtime.]

Translate each of the following signas into clear English:

A. Apply ung. b.i.d.
B. Tab II stat, tab I q 4 h
C. Soak feet qid
D. 1 tab qd hs
E. 1-2 caps q. 8 h.
F. Chart I t.i.d.

————————————————————

A. Apply this ointment twice a day.
B. Take two (2) tablets at once; then take one (1) tablet every four (4) hours.
C. Soak feet four (4) times a day.
D. Take one (1) tablet every day at bedtime.
E. Take one (1) or two (2) capsules every eight (8) hours.
F. Take one (1) powder three (3) times a day.

4. Latin abbreviations often appear in clarifying phrases in the signa. These may indicate whether the medication is to be taken before or after meals, by mouth or some other route of administration, with or without liquids, and so on. Commonly used phrases are given in Table 5–2.

Table 5–2. Selected Latin Abbreviations Used in the Signa

Latin Abbreviation or Term	Meaning
c.	food; meal(s)
a.c.	before meals
p.c.	after meals
c̄, cum	with
s̄, sine	without
rep.	repeat
p.o., per os	by mouth
e.m.p.	in the manner prescribed
ut dict.	as directed
p.r.n.	as needed, when needed

Sometimes, periods are omitted from the abbreviated terms. An example of a signa is

Sig: tab. I p.c. c̄ aq. [Take one (1) tablet after meals with water.]

Translate each of the following signas into clear English.

A. 1 caps t.i.d. a.c. ut. dict.
B. 1 tab c̄ 2 aspirins q 4 h
C. One teaspoonful s̄ aqua; rep. q. 2 h.
D. Rub in prn pain
E. Caps II p.o. p.c. e.m.p.
F. Tab I q.i.d. p.c. & h.s.

––––––––––––––––––––––––––

A. Take one (1) capsule three (3) times a day before meals, as directed.
B. Take one (1) tablet with two (2) aspirin tablets, every four (4) hours.
C. Take one (1) teaspoonful without water. Repeat every two (2) hours.
D. Rub in as needed, to relieve pain.
E. Take two (2) capsules by mouth after meals, in the manner prescribed.
F. Take one (1) tablet four (4) times a day, after meals and at bedtime.

(If these Latin phrases are still Greek to you, review them and try the examples again.)

5. The size of the individual dose may be indicated by the prescriber in terms of the weight or volume of drug that the patient should

obtain. However, directions put on the label for the patient must be written in such a way that they can be understood by the patient. Consider the prescription that follows:

R̟x

    Tetracycline caps   250 mg
Disp. caps. No. XII
Sig: 250 mg q.i.d.

    This prescription calls for 12 capsules, each containing 250 mg of tetracycline. If the directions for use were translated literally as "250 mg four (4) times a day," the patient would not know how many capsules to take. The label should read: "Take one (1) capsule four (4) times a day."

R̟x

    Penicillin V capsules 250 mg
No. 24
Sig: 250 mg q. 4 h 1 h a.c.

How would you write the directions to the patient?

––––––––––––––––––––––––

Take one (1) capsule every four (4) hours, one (1) hour before meals.

---

6.   Consider this prescription:

R̟x

    Sulfisoxazole tabs   0.5 g
Dispense #XLIV
Sig: 2.0 g stat, 1.0 g t.i.d.

A.   How many tablets should be dispensed?
B.   How should the directions to the patient be written?

––––––––––––––––––––––––

A.   44
B.   Take four (4) tablets immediately, then two (2) tablets three (3) times a day.

---

7.   A prescription calls for Penicillin G tablets, each containing 200,000 units. The signa reads "400,000 units q.i.d. for 10 days."

A.   What directions should appear on the label?

B.   How many tablets should be dispensed?

_____

A.   Take two (2) tablets four (4) times a day for ten (10) days.
B.   80 tablets (The patient will use 8 a day for 10 days.)

---

8.   The prescription below is for Mr. Jones. Determine how many days the tablets will last him:

℞

   Sulfadiazine tablets   0.5
d.t.d. No. L
Sig: Tabs II p.c. and h.s.

_____

About 6 days

Solution:

Assuming that the patient eats 3 meals a day, he will take 8 tablets each day. Thus

$$\frac{50 \text{ tab}}{8 \text{ tab/day}} \approx 6 \text{ days}$$

---

9.   To check the safety of a medication, the pharmacist must calculate the dose of each drug being administered to the patient.

℞

   Aspirin   300 mg
   Phenylpropanolamine hydrochloride   20 mg
   Lactose qs ad   600 mg
d.t.d. caps #XXIV
Sig: II q 4 h

   This prescription is for an adult. The usual dose of phenylpropanolamine hydrochloride is listed as "25 to 50 mg every 3 or 4 hours." Calculate the dose of phenylpropanolamine hydrochloride in the prescription and compare it with the usual dose.

_____

Each capsule contains 20 mg of phenylpropanolamine hydrochloride. The patient is therefore taking 40 mg of this drug every 4 hours, which appears to be a satisfactory dose.

10. Consider the following prescription.

℞

Ephedrine sulfate	0.48
Aspirin	7.2
Caffeine	0.24

Div. in caps #XXIV
Sig: Caps II q. 6 h. p.r.n.

How much ephedrine sulfate will the patient be given in each dose, which consists of two capsules?

— — — — — — — — — — — — — — — — — — —

40 mg

Solution:

The quantity of ephedrine sulfate in each capsule may be found by dividing the total quantity of this material by the number of capsules:

$$\frac{480 \text{ mg}}{24 \text{ caps}} = 20 \text{ mg}$$

Thus two capsules will contain 40 mg.

11. Given the following, how many milligrams of hydrocortisone will the patient take each day?

℞

| Hydrocortisone | 0.6 g |
| Sodium salicylate | 30.0 g |

Div. in caps #LX
Sig: caps I q 8 h.

— — — — — — — — — — — — — — — — — — —

30 mg per day. (Each capsule contains 10 mg; 3 capsules are taken each day.)

12. Tablets, capsules, and suppositories are examples of dosage forms that comprise discrete units. When dealing with these unit dosage forms, indication of the size of a dose is a simple matter. The number of units is specified. However, such dosage forms as ointments and solutions are generally dispensed in bulk, and it becomes more difficult to measure dosage accurately.

The dosage of bulk liquids is usually given in terms of household measuring devices such as the teaspoon and tablespoon. There are no uniform, official standards to which teaspoons are made, and a teaspoon found at home may be daintier or heftier than average. According to the official compendia, the average teaspoon holds about 5 mL, but teaspoons in use vary in capacity from about 4 to about 6.5 mL.

In all of our calculations, we will assume that the capacities listed in Table 5–3 are correct. However, to ensure that the patient is actually receiving the intended volume, the pharmacist should give the patient an accurately calibrated measuring device each time that liquid medication is dispensed.

Table 5–3. Household Devices Used to Measure Liquid Medication

Household Measure	Nominal Capacity (mL)
1 teaspoonful	5
1 dessertspoonful	10
1 tablespoonful (1/2 f ʒ)	15
1 glassful (8 f ʒ)	240

The dessertspoonful is used infrequently. It is likely that if a 10-mL dose were required, the patient would be directed to take 2 teaspoonfuls. Note that a teaspoonful is not equivalent to a fluidram (which is closer to 4 mL). A fluidounce contains 8 fluidrams, but only 6 teaspoonfuls.

Learn the table. Then fill in the blanks:

A. 2 f ʒ =   teaspoonfuls.
B. 2 f ʒ =   tablespoonfuls
C. 90 mL =   teaspoonfuls.
D. 120 mL =   tablespoonfuls.
E. 1 tablespoonful =   teaspoonfuls.

————————————————————————

A.   12 teaspoonfuls
B.   4 tablespoonfuls

C.   18 teaspoonfuls
D.   8 tablespoonfuls
E.   3 teaspoonfuls

---

13. Despite the fact that 1 f℥ is not equivalent to 5 mL, when 1 f℥ (or 1 ℥) appears in the signa, it means "1 teaspoonful." In this instance, the symbol has lost its original meaning and should not be interpreted in relation to the apothecary system.

℞

    Elixir terpin hydrate   f℥ IV
Sig: ℥ I t.i.d.

    The directions should read: "Take one (1) teaspoonful three (3) times a day." Since there are 6 teaspoonfuls to a fluidounce, the patient will be given

$$4 \, f℥ \times 6 \text{ teaspoonfuls/} f℥ = 24 \text{ teaspoonfuls}$$

    Each dose consists of 1 teaspoonful, so that 24 doses will be dispensed. This medication will last the patient

$$\frac{24 \text{ doses}}{3 \text{ doses/day}} = 8 \text{ days}$$

For the prescription

℞

    Elixir vit B complex
Disp 180 mL
Sig: f℥ s̅s̅ b.i.d.

the directions should read: "Take one (1) tablespoonful twice a day." A total of

$$180 \text{ mL} \times \frac{1 \text{ tablespoonful}}{15 \text{ mL}} = 12 \text{ tablespoonfuls}$$

will be dispensed. The medication will last the patient

$$\frac{12 \text{ tablespoonfuls}}{2 \text{ tablespoonfuls/day}} = 6 \text{ days}$$

A.   1 ℥ in the signa means _____ .
B.   A fluidounce contains ____ teaspoonfuls or ____ tablespoonfuls.

A.   1 teaspoonful
B.   1 fluidounce = 6 teaspoonfuls = 2 tablespoonfuls

14. Translate each of the following signas into clear English:

A.   ℥ I p.c. c̄ aqua
B.   ℥ I hs
C.   15 mL t.i.d. a.c.
D.   10 mL stat, 5 mL q 6 h

- - - - - - - - - - - - - - - - - - - -

A.   Take one (1) teaspoonful, with water, after meals.
B.   Take two (2) tablespoonfuls at bedtime.
C.   Take one (1) tablespoonful three (3) times a day, before meals.
D.   Take two (2) teaspoonfuls at once, then one (1) teaspoonful every six (6) hours.

15. Given the prescription

℞

    Tetracycline oral syrup

Sig: ℥ s̄s̄ q.i.d. for 6 days

How much tetracycline oral syrup should be dispensed?

- - - - - - - - - - - - - - - - - - - -

60 mL

Solution:

The directions state: "One-half (1/2) teaspoonful four (4) times a day for six (6) days." The patient will therefore take

2 teaspoonfuls/day × 6 days = 12 teaspoonfuls

12 teaspoonfuls × 5 mL/teaspoonful = 60 mL

16. According to the following prescription, how much potassium bromide will the patient be given each day?

R⨯

Potassium bromide	5.4 g
Aqua	30.0 mL
Cherry syrup qs ad	120.0 mL

Sig: 1 teaspoonful qid

- -

0.9 g

Solution:

A total of 4 teaspoonfuls, or 20 mL, of the syrup will be taken each day. The amount of potassium bromide in that quantity can be calculated in several ways. One approach is to set up a proportion, recognizing that the relative content of potassium bromide is the same in any volume of the syrup.

$$\frac{5.4\ \text{g}}{120\ \text{mL}} = \frac{j}{20\ \text{mL}}$$

$j = 0.9$ g

17. The signa for a prescription for 90 mL reads

1 f℥ tid

How many days will this medication last the patient?

- -

6 days

Solution:

$$90.0 \text{ mL} \times \frac{1 \text{ teaspoonful}}{5 \text{ mL}} = 18 \text{ teaspoonfuls in the bottle}$$

$$\frac{18 \text{ teaspoonfuls}}{3 \text{ teaspoonfuls/day}} = 6 \text{ days}$$

18. ℞

Chlorpheniramine maleate syrup
Disp 3-day supply
Sig: 4 mg b.i.d.

Each 5 mL of this syrup contains 2 mg of chlorpheniramine maleate.

A.   What directions for use should be put on the label?
B.   How much chlorpheniramine maleate syrup should be dispensed?

_ _

A.   Take two (2) teaspoonfuls twice a day.
B.   60 mL should be dispensed.

Solution:

Each 5 mL of syrup = 2 mg of drug. The patient takes 8 mg per day, or 24 mg during the three-day period.

$$24 \text{ mg} \times \frac{5 \text{ mL}}{2 \text{ mg}} = 60 \text{ mL of syrup}$$

19. ℞

Milk of bismuth   15.0
dtd #6
Sig: 15 mL ut dict

A.   What are the directions to the patient?
B.   What quantity of milk of bismuth should be dispensed?

A.   Take one (1) tablespoonful as directed.
B.   15 mL × 6 = 90 mL

20. Here are some practice problems dealing with dosage calculations
     in prescriptions.

A.   ℞

         Elixir phenobarbital   30 mL
         Lactated pepsin elix   30 mL
         Syrup tolu qs ad   120 mL
     Sig: 1 teaspoonful tid ac

     How many doses will the patient get?

B.   ℞
         Donnagel PG
     Sig: f ʒ ss t.i.d. p.c. c̄ aq.

     (1) What directions would you put on the label?
     (2) How many milliliters of Donnagel PG should be dispensed so
         as to last the patient 4 days?

C.   ℞
         Syrup Phenergan
     Sig: ʒ I qid, pc & hs

     How many milliliters of syrup Phenergan should be dispensed if
     this prescription is to last the patient six days?

D. ℞

        Ampicillin syrup (125 mg/teaspoonful)

Sig: 250 mg qid for 10 days

How many milliliters of this syrup will the patient take all together?

E. ℞

Ammonium chloride	8 g
Benylin expectorant	40 mL
Water qs ad	120 mL

How many milligrams of ammonium chloride does each teaspoonful of the prescription contain?

F. ℞

Sodium bromide	3 g
Lactose qs ad	5 g

Div in caps #24

Sig: Caps II tid

Calculate the total daily dose of sodium bromide.

G. ℞

Ephedrine sulfate syrup	60.0
Chlortrimeton syrup	60.0

   M

Sig: ʒ I q.i.d.

How many days will this quantity of medication last the patient?

H.   ℞

      Benadryl caps   50 mg
No. 30
Sig: Caps I a.c., caps II h.s.

How many days will this prescription last the patient?

I.   ℞

      Ferrous gluconate   1.5 g
      Ascorbic acid   15.0 g
Div. in caps No. 96
Sig: caps I b.i.d.

In how many days will the patient have ingested 280 mg of ferrous gluconate?

J.   ℞

      PBZ expectorant   90 mL
      Ephedrine syrup   90 mL
Sig: 1 tablespoonful tid

How many days will this prescription last the patient?

K. ℞

       Ammonium bromide   10 g

       Syrup   20 mL

       Peppermint water qs ad 120 mL

    Sig: ℥ I qid

How many milligrams of ammonium bromide does the patient take each day?

- - - - - - - - - - - - - - - - - - -

A. 24

B. (1) 1 tablespoonful 3 times a day after meals, with water

    (2) 180 mL

C. 120 mL

D. 400 mL

E. 333 mg

F. 0.75 g

G. 6 days

H. 6 days

I. 9 days

J. 4 days

K. 1670 mg

21. Liquid medication intended for use in the eye, ear, or nose is usually dispensed in a dropper bottle. The patient is directed to measure the dose by counting drops. The Latin abbreviations listed in Table 5–4 are frequently used.

Table 5–4. Abbreviations for Signa of Liquids Administered by Drop

Latin Abbreviation	Meaning
gtt	drop
o.d.	right eye
o.s.	left eye
o.u.	both eyes

Translate these signas into clear English:

A. 2 gtt o.s. q.d.

B.   Gtt. I o.u. b.i.d.

       _____

A.   Put two (2) drops in the left eye once a day.
B.   Put one (1) drop in both eyes twice a day.

---

22.   Sometimes, the dose of a liquid intended for oral administration is
      too small to be measured with a teaspoon. Use of a calibrated
      dropper may solve the problem. By knowing the volume of each
      drop, the number of drops of a liquid necessary to make up the
      desired dose can be calculated. The volume of a drop depends
      upon the size of the dropper orifice and the viscosity and surface
      tension of the liquid, among other factors. It is therefore
      necessary to calibrate the dropper for use with the specific liquid
      that will be dispensed. This is accomplished by counting the
      number of drops that exactly equal a definite volume (2.0 mL or
      more using a 10-mL graduate since less than 20% of the capacity
      should not be measured).
            This calibration provides us with a statement of equivalence
      between milliliters and "drops" as a measure of volume. For
      example, a solution for administration to a child was prepared.
      The dose of the solution was 1.2 mL. (A dose measuring 1/4
      teaspoonful would be a very inaccurate way of administering the
      solution.) A dropper calibrated with the solution delivered 2.0 mL
      in 44 drops. We may therefore write

           2.0 mL = 44 drops

or

           1.0 mL = 22 drops

The number of drops equivalent to 1.2 mL is

$$1.2 \text{ mL} \times \frac{22 \text{ drops}}{1.0 \text{ mL}} = 26 \text{ drops}$$

      A dropper was found to deliver 3.0 mL of saline solution in 75
drops. If 14 drops were put in a test tube, how many cubic
centimeters of saline solution did the test tube contain?

————————————————————

0.56 cc

Solution:

3.0 mL = 75 drops

$$14 \text{ drops} \times \frac{3.0 \text{ mL}}{75 \text{ drops}} = 0.56 \text{ mL} = 0.56 \text{ cc}$$

---

23. A prescription has 0.4 mL of peppermint oil as one of its ingredients. A dropper was calibrated and found to deliver 2.0 mL of peppermint oil in 55 drops. How many drops of peppermint oil should be used?

————————————————————

11 drops

Solution:

2.0 mL

$$0.4 \text{ mL} \times \frac{55 \text{ drops}}{2.0 \text{ mL}} = 11 \text{ drops}$$

---

24. In the hospital, patients often receive solutions intravenously (directly into a vein). It may be necessary to administer a large volume of solution. This is done slowly, over a period of time, using a device that can be adjusted to deliver a chosen number of drops per minute. The process is called *intravenous infusion*.

    Here is a typical problem: A patient is to receive 900 mL of a solution over 12 hours (h). If 20 drops = 1 mL, at how many drops/min should the medication be infused?

    From the information given, we can calculate the number of mL/min that must be administered. Then, by converting milliliters to drops, it will be possible to determine the number of drops/min.

$$\frac{900 \text{ mL}}{12 \text{ h}} = 75 \text{ mL/h}$$

$$75 \text{ mL/h} \times \frac{1 \text{ h}}{60 \text{ min}} = 1.25 \text{ mL/min}$$

$$1.25 \text{ mL/min} \times 20 \text{ drops/mL} = 25 \text{ drops/min}$$

A solution is to be administered by intravenous infusion at a rate of 45 mL/h. How many drops/min should be infused if 1 mL = 40 drops?

- -

30 drops/min

Solution:

$$45 \text{ mL/h} \times \frac{1 \text{ h}}{60 \text{ min}} = 0.75 \text{ mL/min}$$

$$0.75 \text{ mL/min} \times 40 \text{ drops/mL} = 30 \text{ drops/min}$$

25. A patient is to receive 2000 mL of a solution by intravenous infusion over a period of 24 h. What rate of infusion (drops/min) should be utilized if 1 mL = 20 drops?

- -

28 drops/min

Solution:

$$\frac{2000 \text{ mL}}{24 \text{ h}} = 83.3 \text{ mL/h}$$

$$83.3 \text{ mL/h} \times \frac{1 \text{ h}}{60 \text{ min}} \times \frac{20 \text{ drops}}{1 \text{ mL}} = 27.8 \text{ drops/min}$$

This may be rounded off to 28 drops/min.

26. A patient receives a solution by intravenous infusion at a rate of 36 drops/min. How much solution is infused in 3 h if 1 mL = 30 drops?

_____

216 mL

Solution:

$$36 \text{ drops/min} \times \frac{1 \text{ mL}}{30 \text{ drops}} = 1.2 \text{ mL/min}$$

$$1.2 \text{ mL/min} \times 180 \text{ min} = 216 \text{ mL}$$

27. One hundred micrograms of a drug, dissolved in 240 mL of solution, is to be infused at a rate of 25 µg/h. If 1 mL = 15 drops, what should the rate of administration be (in drops/min)?

_____

15 drops/min

If you were able to handle this problem, continue with frame 31. If you had trouble, go to the next frame.

28. Remember that our calculations deal with flow rates. We know that the drug has to be infused at a rate of 25 µg/h. We have to first determine the rate of infusion, in mL/h, for the solution that contains the drug. Knowing that each 240 mL holds 100 µg of drug, find the volume that contains 25 µg. This is the volume that must be administered each hour. Then see if you can complete the solution.

The volume of solution to be infused each hour can be found by proportion.

$$\frac{100 \ \mu g}{240 \ mL} = \frac{25 \ \mu g}{j}$$

$j = 60 \ mL$

$$60 \ mL/h \times \frac{1 \ h}{60 \ min} \times \frac{15 \ drops}{1 \ mL} = 15 \ drops/min$$

---

29. A solution for intravenous infusion contains 0.025 µg/mL of a drug. Calculate the flow rate, in drops/min, needed to administer the drug at a rate of 2 µg/h. 1 mL = 25 drops.

---

33 drops/min

Solution:

$$\frac{0.025 \ \mu g}{1 \ mL} = \frac{2 \ \mu g}{j}$$

$j = 80 \ mL$

$$80 \ mL/h \times \frac{1 \ h}{60 \ min} \times 25 \ drops/mL = 33 \ drops/min$$

---

30. You can do these problems for additional practice.

A. A dropper delivers 4.0 mL of caraway oil in 110 drops. How many drops will deliver 1.3 mL?

B. ℞

>   Opium tincture   0.3 mL
>   Cascara sagrada fluid extract   2.0 mL
>   Syrup tolu qs ad   5.0 mL
>   Ft sol dtd #12

A dropper, calibrated with opium tincture, delivers 1.0 mL in 33 drops. How many drops of opium tincture should be used to fill this prescription?

C. ℞

>   Paregoric   1.5 mL
>   Milk of bismuth qs ad   5.0 mL
>   d.t.d. No. 6
>   Sig: 20 drops a.c.

If the dropper dispensed with this prescription delivers 2.0 mL in 26 drops, how many milliliters of paregoric are in each dose?

D. Fifteen hundred milliliters of a solution is to be administered to a patient by intravenous infusion over a period of 24 h. At what rate, in drops/min, should the solution be given if 1 mL = 25 drops?

E. A solution contains 1.25 mg of a drug per milliliter. At what rate should the solution be infused (drops/min) if the drug is to be administered at a rate of 80 mg/h? 1 mL = 30 drops.

A. 36 drops
B. 119 drops
C. 0.462 mL
D. 26 drops/min
E. 32 drops/min

---

31. The usual adult dose of a drug is that quantity which is expected to exert the desired effect in most adults. A valuable reference for the pharmacist in checking prescribed doses is Volume I of the USP DI. This publication contains a compilation of useful drug information directed primarily to health care professionals. Individual drug descriptions, called monographs, contain such information as the therapeutic category, pharmacology, precautions, and side effects in addition to dosing information.

Young children (pediatrics) and older people (geriatrics) often require special consideration because their excretion and metabolism of certain drugs may differ significantly from the way these drugs are handled by the standard adult population. In fact, many adults vary in size from what is considered the norm and the dose may have to be adjusted for them. For guidance with respect to dosing of children, the usual pediatric dose listed in the USP DI is a valuable reference. Another useful source of information is the Pediatric Dosage Handbook published by the American Pharmaceutical Association.

There are a number of ways for making dosage adjustments to suit individual requirements. The most accurate are based on data obtained from testing performed on the patient. This is especially valuable (and cost-effective) for highly potent drugs with a narrow margin of safety.

Sometimes dosage adjustment is accomplished by expressing the dose as a quantity of drug per unit weight of the patient. The dose, determined in this way, is usually calculated to two significant figures.

The usual dose of diethylcarbamazine citrate is 2 mg per kilogram of body weight, three times a day for 1 to 3 weeks. The dose for a particular person is determined by his or her weight in kilograms. For an 80-kg adult, the dose is

$$2 \text{ mg/kg} \times 80 \text{ kg} = 160 \text{ mg}$$

The daily dose of a drug is 12 µg per kilogram of body weight. How many milligrams should be administered each day to a woman who weighs 55 kg?

0.66 mg

Solution:

$$55 \text{ kg} \times 12 \text{ µg/kg} = 660 \text{ µg} = 0.66 \text{ mg}$$

32. If the dose of a drug is 0.25 mg/kg, how many milligrams should be administered to a man weighing 175 lb?

----

20 mg

Solution:

$$175 \text{ lb} \times \frac{1 \text{ kg}}{2.20 \text{ lb}} \times 0.25 \text{ mg/kg} = 20 \text{ mg}$$

33. The usual dose of lucanthone hydrochloride is 5.0 mg per kilogram of body weight three times a day for 1 week. What should the total daily dose, in grams, be for a youth weighing 120 lb?

0.81 g

Solution:

$$120 \text{ lb} \times \frac{1 \text{ kg}}{2.20 \text{ lb}} \times 5 \text{ mg/kg} = 270 \text{ mg}$$

Since 3 doses are administered each day, the total will be 810 mg or 0.81 g.

34. Instead of body weight, body surface area may be used to estimate the dose for a patient. This is considered to be more accurate in many cases. The average adult weighs 150 lb and has a body surface area of 1.73 m^2.

   The dose of a drug is 200 mg/m^2. What is the dose for a child whose body surface area is 0.8 m^2?

———————————————————

160 mg

Solution:

$$200 \text{ mg/m}^2 \times 0.8 \text{ m}^2 = 160 \text{ mg}$$

35. The dose of a drug is 15 mg/m^2, twice a day, for 1 week. How many milligrams of the drug should the patient take altogether in the course of treatment? Assume that the patient is an average adult.

———————————————————

364 mg

Solution:

Each dose should be

$$15.0 \text{ mg/m}^2 \times 1.73 \text{ m}^2 = 26 \text{ mg}$$

Since the drug is given b.i.d. for 1 week, a total of 14 doses will be administered:

$$26 \text{ mg} \times 14 = 364 \text{ mg}$$

---

36. One of the difficulties in calculating dosage on the basis of body surface area is the necessity for first estimating the patient's surface area. Various tables and graphs that relate body surface area to more easily measured things such as the patient's weight and height have been published. Separate nomographs for adults and children have been computed and are available for use by the physician and pharmacist. For children of average height, the surface area may be estimated from the formula

$$S = \frac{4w + 7}{w + 90}$$

where S is surface area in square meters and w is the weight in kilograms.
    Using the formula, estimate the body surface area of a child weighing

A. 10 kg
B. 30 kg

A. 0.47 m^2
B. 1.1 m^2

---

37. The formula given in frame 38 is useful for checking, at least in an approximate fashion, prescribed doses for children. For example, the usual pediatric (child's) dose of pyrvinium, a drug used to treat intestinal pinworms, is 150 mg per square meter of

body surface, administered as a single dose. Let us say that pyrvinium is administered to a child weighing 15 kg. According to the formula,

$$S = \frac{60 + 7}{15 + 90} = \frac{67}{105} = 0.64 \text{ m}^2$$

$$0.64 \text{ m}^2 \times 150 \text{ mg/m}^2 = 96 \text{ mg}$$

The child's dose should be approximately 96 mg. If the prescribed dose is close to this value, fine. If not, the pharmacist should check further before dispensing the medication.

---

38. The approximate equation utilized in the previous frames may not be accurate enough when dealing with very short or tall children. More accurate computations utilize both weight and height measurements. The following equations are given in the Pediatric Dosage Handbook:

$$S = \sqrt{\frac{I \times P}{3131}}$$

$$S = \sqrt{\frac{C \times K}{3600}}$$

In the first equation, I is height in inches and P the weight in pounds. In the second equation, C is height in centimeters and K weight in kilograms. Although nomograms are available to simplify determination of body surface area, the equations are easy enough to use with the aid of a calculator.
    A 44-pound child has a height of 40 inches. Calculate the body surface area from
A.   the approximate equation given in frame 36.
B.   either of the more exact equations in this frame.

- -

A.   0.79 m^2
B.   0.75 m^2

39. Do all of the problems in this frame before verifying your answers.

A. Write each of these signas so that a patient would understand them:

   (1) Tab I q 4 h prn

   (2) 5.0 mL c̄ aq. p.c. h.s.

   (3) Gtt. II o.s. b.i.d.

   (4) Apply ung qd ut dict

   (5) ℥ s̅s̅ s̄ aq. t.i.d.

   (6) Gtt. x p.o. a.c.

B. ℞

       Amphetamine sulfate   90 mg
       Lactose qs
   Div in caps No XX

       How many milligrams of amphetamine sulfate will each capsule contain?

C. ℞

       Ephedrine sulfate syrup   60 mL
       Dimetane syrup   120 mL
   M
   Sig: 2 teasp t.i.d.

       How many days will this prescription last the patient?

D.   ℞

   Cinnamon water   1.5 mL
   Sodium phenobarbital 0.015 g
   Aromatic elixir qs ad 5.0 mL
 d.t.d. No. 24
 Sig: 13 q.i.d. a.c.

  How much sodium phenobarbital should be used for this prescription? How many milligrams of sodium phenobarbital will the patient receive each day?

E.   ℞

   Milk of bismuth
 Sig: 1 tablespoonful tid

  How many fluid ounces should be dispensed if the bottle is to last the patient 4 days?

F.   ℞

   Elixophyllin
 Dispense 1 pint
 Sig: 1 tablespoon t.i.d.

  If the patient stops using this medication after seven days, how many fluidounces of Elixophyllin will be left in the bottle?

G.   ℞

   Penicillin V suspension 240 mL
   (each teaspoonful contains 200,000 units)
 Sig: 400,000 units t.i.d.

How many days will this prescription last the patient?

H.   ℞

       Hydrocortisone   0.45 g
       Sodium salicylate   30 g
Div. in caps. No. LX
Sig: caps II q. 12 h. p.c.

How many milligrams of hydrocortisone will the patient take each day?

I.   ℞

       Sodium pentobarbital   5 gr
       Orange syrup   30 mL
       Syrup qs ad   90 mL

How many milligrams of sodium pentobarbital does each teaspoonful contain?

J.   ℞

       Papaverine hydrochloride   1.0 g
       Aqua   30.0 mL
       Syrup tolu q.s. ad   90.0 mL
Sig: f ℥ I t.i.d.

How many milligrams of papaverine will the patient receive each day?

K. ℞

          Sodium pentobarbital   0.090 g
          Cherry syrup qs ad   30 mL
     Sig: 10 mg of sod. pentobarb. h.s.

     If the dropper dispensed with the product delivers 2.0 mL in 48 drops, how many drops would contain 10 mg of sodium pentobarbital?

L. Five hundred milligrams of an antibiotic are dissolved in 100 mL of a solution to be administered by intravenous infusion. What should the drop rate be (in drops/min) if 1 mL = 15 drops and the antibiotic is to be given over a period of 1 h?

M. The dose of a drug is 250 μg/kg of body weight. How many milligrams should be administered to a 175-lb man?

N. The dose of a drug is 0.6 mg per square meter of body surface area. How many micrograms should be administered to a child whose body surface area is 0.75 m^2?

O. The usual pediatric dose of a drug is 12 μg/m^2. Calculate the dose for a child weighing 35 pounds whose height is 32 inches.

_ _

A. (1) Take one (1) tablet every four (4) hours as needed.
    (2) Take one (1) teaspoonful with water after meals and at bedtime.
    (3) Put two (2) drops in the left eye twice a day.
    (4) Apply this ointment every day as directed.
    (5) Take one (1) tablespoonful without water three (3) times a day.
    (6) Take ten (10) drops by mouth before meals.
B. 4.5 mg
C. 6 days
D. 360 mg should be used; 60 mg per day
E. 6 f ʒ
F. 5 1/2 f ʒ
G. 8 days
H. 30 mg
I. 18 mg
J. 167 mg
K. 80 drops
L. 25 drops/min
M. 20 mg
N. 450 µg
O. 7.2 µg

Solutions:

A. Shown above.

B. $\dfrac{90 \text{ mg}}{20 \text{ caps}} = 4.5 \text{ mg/caps}$

C. The total volume dispensed is 180 mL. Each day, the patient takes 6 teaspoonfuls, or 30 mL:

$$\dfrac{180 \text{ mL}}{30 \text{ mL/day}} = 6 \text{ days}$$

D. sodium phenobarbital: 15 mg/teasp × 24 teasp = 360 mg

daily dose: 15 mg/teasp × 4 teasp/day = 60 mg/day

E. 0.5 f ʒ/dose × 3 doses/day = 1.5 f ʒ/day

4 days × 1.5 f ʒ/day = 6 f ʒ

F.   The patient takes 3 tablespoonfuls, or 1.5 f℥, each day:

7 days × 1.5 f℥/day = 10.5 f℥ used

16 f℥ – 10.5 f℥ = 5.5 f℥ remain

G.   400,000 units = 2 teaspoonfuls

The patient takes 2 teaspoonfuls three times a day, for a total of 6 teaspoonfuls or 30 mL.

$$\frac{240 \text{ mL}}{30 \text{ mL/day}} = 8 \text{ days}$$

H.   Four capsules are taken each day.

$$\frac{450 \text{ mg}}{60 \text{ caps}} \times 4 \text{ caps/day} = 30 \text{ mg/day}$$

I. $$\frac{5 \text{ gr}}{90 \text{ mL}} = \frac{j}{5 \text{ mL}}$$

$j = 0.28$ gr

0.28 gr × 64.8 mg/gr = 18 mg

J.   The total daily amount taken is 15 mL

$$\frac{1000 \text{ mg}}{90 \text{ mL}} = \frac{j}{15 \text{ mL}}$$

$j = 167$ mg

K. $$\frac{90 \text{ mg}}{30 \text{ mL}} = \frac{10 \text{ mg}}{j}$$

$j = 3.33$ mL

$$3.33 \text{ mL} \times \frac{48 \text{ drops}}{2 \text{ mL}} = 80 \text{ drops}$$

L. $$\frac{100 \text{ mL}}{1 \text{ h}} \times \frac{1 \text{ h}}{60 \text{ min}} \times 15 \text{ drops/mL} = 25 \text{ drops/min}$$

M. $$175 \text{ lb} \times \frac{1 \text{ kg}}{2.20 \text{ lb}} \times 0.25 \text{ mg/kg} = 20 \text{ mg}$$

N. $0.75 \text{ m}^2 \times 600 \text{ µg/m}^2 = 450 \text{ µg}$

O. $S = \sqrt{\dfrac{I \times P}{3131}} = \sqrt{\dfrac{32 \times 35}{3131}} = 0.60 \text{ m}^2$

$0.6 \text{ m}^2 \times 12 \text{ μg/m}^2 = 7.2 \text{ μg}$

CHAPTER SIX

PERCENTAGE STRENGTH

Up to this point we have dealt with prescriptions and formulas in which quantities of the ingredients have been expressed as weights or volumes. Some formulas specify the concentrations of the ingredients used, usually as a percent. Other indications of concentration, such as parts per million and parts per billion are useful in describing very dilute solutions..

Learning objectives: after completing this chapter the student should be able to

1. State the meaning of weight in weight, volume in volume and weight in volume systems.
2. Apply the default rules that decide which system type is indicated in the absence of a specific designation.
3. Calculate quantities needed to weigh or measure ingredients in prescriptions or other formulas written on the basis of percent.
4. Determine concentration from the quantities used in a preparation.
5. Determine the amount of solvent needed for a liquid preparation from weight designations or liquid volume and density.
6. Perform calculations in which concentration is specified as parts per million or parts per billion.

---

1. Expressions of concentration describe the amount of solute that will be contained in some definite quantity of the total preparation. If sodium chloride is dissolved in water, the

---

concentration of the solution is characterized by the weight of sodium chloride dissolved and the volume of solution (not solvent). We may define concentration thus:

$$\text{concentration} = \frac{\text{quantity of solute}}{\text{quantity of preparation}}$$

Concentration is dependent upon the quantity of solute and the quantity of _____ .

_ _

solution or preparation

2. If the solute and the preparation are expressed in the same units, the concentration is dimensionless. It indicates the portion of the preparation represented by solute, and is written as a decimal or fraction. For example, if 10.0 mL of alcohol were dissolved in a sufficient quantity of water to make 40.0 mL of solution, the concentration of alcohol would be

$$\frac{10.0 \text{ mL}}{40.0 \text{ mL}} = 0.250$$

Percent concentration is defined as the number of parts of solute in 100 units of solution. Concentration expressed as a decimal may be converted to percent by multiplying by 100:

$$0.250 \times 100 = 25.0\%$$

This concentration may be written 25.0% by volume or 25.0% volume in volume or 25.0% v/v to indicate that both the solute and solution were measured by volume.

3. If 12.0 mL of peppermint oil were dissolved in sufficient alcohol to make 80.0 mL of solution, what would be the concentration of peppermint oil in this solution expressed as

A. a decimal?
B. a percent?

_ _

A.   0.150 v/v
B.   15.0% v/v

Solutions:

A.   concentration $= \dfrac{12.0 \text{ mL}}{80.0 \text{ mL}} = 0.150$ v/v

B. $0.150 \text{ v/v} \times 100 = 15.0\%$ v/v

---

4.   If the quantity of solute and of the preparation are expressed in the same units of weight, the concentration is dimensionless. If 10.0 g of charcoal are mixed with 65.0 g of another powder to make a total of 75.0 g, the charcoal concentration is

$$\frac{10.0 \text{ g}}{75.0 \text{ g}} = 0.133 \text{ by weight (or 13.3\% w/w)}$$

In a preparation in which all concentrations are w/w, the sum of all contributions must be 100%.
    If 12.0 g of lanolin are combined with 2.0 g of white wax and 16.0 g of petrolatum to make an ointment, what is the percentage concentration of lanolin in the ointment?

_ _

40.0% w/w

Solution:
$$\frac{12.0 \text{ g lanolin}}{30.0 \text{ g ointment}} = 0.400 = 40.0\% \text{ w/w}$$

---

5.   When the solute is measured by weight and the solution by volume, concentration is not dimensionless. If 1.25 g of sodium chloride are dissolved in sufficient water to make 55.0 mL of solution, the concentration is

$$\frac{1.25 \text{ g}}{55.0 \text{ mL}} = 0.0227 \text{ g/mL}$$

Commonly, this concentration will be stated as a percent, w/v. The appendage "w/v" tells us that the solute is expressed in grams and that the quantity of solution is determined by volume in milliliters. These implied units must not be neglected in calculations.

By multiplying grams per milliliter by 100, we obtain the number of grams in 100 mL, which defines percent w/v:

$$0.0227 \text{ g/mL} = \frac{2.27 \text{ g}}{100 \text{ mL}} = 2.27\% \text{ w/v}$$

---

6.   If 5.75 g of boric acid are dissolved in sufficient alcohol to make a total volume of 120 mL, what is the strength of boric acid in the solution in

A.   g/mL?
B.   percent w/v?

– –

A. $\dfrac{5.75 \text{ g}}{120 \text{ mL}} = 0.0479 \text{ g/mL}$
B. $0.0479 \text{ g/mL} \times 100 = 4.79\% \text{ w/v}$

---

7.   To review these definitions of percent, the concentration of substance in a solution or mixture is expressed in terms of the amount of substance and the finished preparation. If the concentration is p percent w/w, then 100 weight units of the preparation contain p weight units of substance. The same weight units must be used for both substance and preparation. If the concentration is q percent v/v, then 100 volume units of the preparation contain q volume units of substance. The same volume units are used for both substance and preparation. If the concentration is r percent w/v, then 100 mL of the preparation contain r grams of substance.

In each case, determine the percent concentration of glycerin and indicate whether w/w, v/v, or w/v:

A.   4.00 g of glycerin are dissolved in sufficient alcohol to make 25.0 mL.

B.   1.50 g of phenol are dissolved in 8.00 g of glycerin.

C.   10.0 mL of glycerin are dissolved in sufficient water to make 38.0 mL of solution.

- -

A.   16.0% w/v
B.   84.2% w/w
C.   26.3% v/v

Solutions:

A. $\dfrac{4.00 \text{ g}}{25.0 \text{ mL}}$ = 0.160 g/mL = 16.0% w/v

B. $\dfrac{8.00 \text{ g}}{9.50 \text{ g}}$ = 0.842 w/w = 84.2% w/w

C. $\dfrac{10.0 \text{ mL}}{38.0 \text{ mL}}$ = 0.263 v/v = 26.3% v/v

8.   Sometimes the concentration of a solution is indicated without stating whether it is to be w/w, w/v, or v/v. In such cases, solutions are prepared so that solids can be weighed and liquids measured by volume. When the solute and the solvent (and therefore the solution) are liquids, the solution strength is assumed to be percent v/v. If the solute is a solid and the solvent a liquid, solution strength is assumed to be percent w/v. If both the solute and solvent are solid (or in a mixture of solids) percent w/w is assumed. These default rules come into play only when the percentage type is not indicated.

Let us look at an example. Say that you make up a solution of peppermint oil in alcohol by dissolving 2.0 mL of oil in enough alcohol to make 100 mL of solution. The concentration is

$$\frac{2.0 \text{ mL}}{100 \text{ mL}} = 0.02 \text{ v/v} = 2.0\% \text{ v/v}$$

If your product is labeled "Peppermint Oil Solution, 2.0%," the default rules apply. Since both peppermint oil and alcohol are liquids, it is assumed that both will be measured by volume. Therefore, "2.0%" means 2.0% v/v in this case, so that your label describes the product accurately.

But what if you were to make up a solution by dissolving 2.0 g of peppermint oil in sufficient alcohol to make up 100 mL of solution? Then "2.0%" would not accurately describe the product. It would have to be labeled 2.0% w/v.

If 4.0 g of peppermint oil are dissolved in 96.0 g of alcohol, how would you describe the concentration of peppermint oil in this solution? If you think that the answer is

A.   4.0%, go to frame 11.
B.   4.0% v/v, go to frame 10.
C.   4.0% w/w, go to frame 12.
D.   4.0% w/v, go to frame 9.

---

9.   A concentration of "4.0% w/v" means that 4.0 g of peppermint oil are present in 100 mL of solution. That is not the way this solution was made up. Go back to frame 8 and try again.

---

10. A concentration of "4.0% v/v" means that 4.0 mL of peppermint oil are present in 100 mL of solution. That is not the way this solution was made up. Go back to frame 8 and try again.

---

11. Since peppermint oil and alcohol are liquids, "4.0%" means that 4.0 mL of peppermint oil are present in 100 mL of solution. But this solution was not made up by volume, so that the default rules cannot be used. Read frame 8 over carefully, and then see if you can answer the question correctly.

---

12. You are correct. Peppermint oil and alcohol are liquids and would normally be measured by volume. But in this example, the solution was prepared by weight. The "percent w/w" designation transmits this information. If the concentration were written "4.0%," the default rules would apply and we would be

(incorrectly) led to believe that the solution was prepared by volume.

---

13. Decide whether each of the following systems is w/w, v/v, or w/v, using the default rules:

A. 1% solution of zinc sulfate (a solid) in distilled water
B. An ointment containing 3% sulfur in petrolatum (both solids)
C. 10% solution of sugar in alcohol
D. 15% solution of alcohol in distilled water

_____

A. w/v
B. w/w
C. w/v
D. v/v

---

14. In a moment we will work with some prescriptions in which the ingredients are listed by percent. Of course, in order to prepare the medication, it is necessary to convert the percentages to weights and volumes. In w/w prescriptions, we calculate the weight of each material, since each must be weighed individually. But in w/v and v/v solutions, the volume of the solvent is usually not determined explicitly. There are two reasons:

First, the solution is usually completed in a graduate by adding sufficient solvent to make the desired final volume. It is thus not necessary to know the volume of solvent.

Second, it is often impossible to calculate exactly what the volume of solvent should be. In w/v solutions, the volume occupied by the dissolved solute is not known. In very dilute solutions, the volume of solute may be negligible. But in general, there is no way to tell how much solvent to use.

In v/v solutions, there may be shrinkage of volume when certain liquids are mixed: 50 mL of alcohol plus 50 mL of water yield less than 100 mL of solution. However, when chemically similar liquids are combined (e.g., mixing one fixed oil with another or one hydrocarbon with another), the total volume is usually the sum of the volumes of the components.

---

15. ℞

Zinc sulfate (a solid)	1/2%
Aq. pur. qs ad	60.0 mL

In this prescription the drug content is specified on the basis of concentration. We must calculate the quantities needed to prepare this solution. Zinc sulfate is a solid and the final product is a liquid, so the concentration is taken to be w/v. Thus the zinc sulfate concentration is 0.5 g/100 mL or 0.005 g/mL.

The most direct way of calculating the quantity of zinc sulfate is to rearrange the definition of concentration:

$$\text{concentration} = \frac{\text{quantity of solute}}{\text{quantity of solution}}$$

quantity of solute = quantity of solution × concentration

0.005 g/mL × 60.0 mL = 0.3 g

Dissolve 0.3 g of zinc sulfate in sufficient purified water to make 60 mL.

Now consider this prescription:

℞

| Eucalyptus oil | 2.5% v/v |
| Mineral oil qs ad | 30.0 |

What quantities should be used for this prescription?

- - - - - - - - - - - - - - - - - - - -

Eucalyptus oil: 0.750 mL
Mineral oil: sufficient to make 30.0 mL of solution

Solution:

30.0 mL × 0.025 = 0.75 mL

---

16. ℞

Sulfur	10.0%
Benzoic acid	1.5%
Petrolatum qs ad	30.0
Ft ung	

All ingredients are solids. What quantity of each should be used to make this ointment? (Remember that all three ingredients must be weighed.)

_____

Sulfur: 3.00 g
Benzoic acid: 0.450 g
Petrolatum: 26.6 g

Solution:

All ingredients are solids. According to the default rules, we treat the concentrations as percent w/w:

Sulfur: 30.0 g × 0.1 = 3.00 g

Benzoic acid: 30.0 g × 0.015 = 0.450 g

The sum of all percentages must be 100%. This is necessarily true only in a preparation in which all concentrations are w/w. From the prescription, we can see that 88.5% of the ointment is petrolatum.

Petrolatum: 30 0 g × 0.885 = 26.6 g

To check, verify that the sum of all contributions is 30.0 g.

---

17. ℞

Boric acid	2%
Camphor water	35%
Aqua pur qs ad	15.0 mL

Ft. sol

How much boric acid (a solid) and camphor water (a liquid) are needed for this prescription? (Here is a situation in which two concentration types appear in the same solution. The boric acid must be considered on a w/v basis, whereas the camphor water is handled on a v/v basis. Treat each substance separately in doing your calculations.)

Boric acid: 300 mg
Camphor water: 5.25 mL

Solution:

    Boric acid: 15.0 mL × 0.02 g/mL = 0.300 g

    Camphor water: 15.0 mL × 0.35 = 5.25 mL

18. Now try these.

A.   R

        Menthol   0.8%
        Alcohol qs ad   60.0 mL

    Menthol is a solid. How many grams should be used to
    prepare this prescription?

B.   R

        Zinc oxide
        Talc $\overline{aa}$ 15%
        Lanolin
        Petrolatum $\overline{aa}$ qs ad   60 g

    All ingredients are solids. Calculate the weight of each
    ingredient needed.

C. What quantity of each ingredient in the following prescription
    should be used? Include units.

℞

Ammonium chloride (solid)   5%
Syrup tolu (liquid)   35%
Syrup wild cherry qs ad   120 mL

_____

A. 0.48 g
B. Zinc oxide: 9 g
    Talc: 9 g
    Lanolin: 21 g
    Petrolatum: 21 g
C. Ammonium chloride: 6 g
    Syrup tolu: 42 mL
    Syrup wild cherry: qs to make 120 mL

---

19. Iodine tincture is a 2% w/v solution of iodine.

A. How many grams of iodine will 40.0 mL of the tincture contain?

B. How many milliliters of the tincture contain 0.600 g of iodine?
    (Use proportion or rearrange the concentration definition to solve
    for amount of preparation.)

_____

A. 0.8 g
B. 30.0 mL

Solutions:

A.   40.0 mL × 0.02 g/mL = 0.8 g

B. $\dfrac{2\ g}{100\ mL} = \dfrac{0.6\ g}{j}$

   $j = 30$ mL

Alternatively,

$$\text{amount of preparation} = \frac{\text{amount of solute}}{\text{concentration}}$$

$$\frac{0.6\ g}{2\ g/100\ mL} = 30\ mL$$

---

20. How many liters of a 0.9% aqueous solution can be made from 20.0 g of sodium chloride?

- -

2.22 L

Solution:

$$\frac{0.9\ g}{100\ mL} = \frac{20.0\ g}{j}$$

   $j = 2220$ mL = 2.22 L

---

21. Try these problems for additional practice.

A.   Diluted hydrochloric acid is a 10% w/v solution of HCl in water. How many milligrams of HCl does each teaspoonful of diluted hydrochloric acid contain?

B. How many milliliters of a 6.70% v/v solution contain 850 µL of solute?

C. How many liters of a 2.50% w/v solution can be prepared using 42.5 g of solute?

D. A boric acid preparation contains:

Boric acid: 2 parts by weight
Liquid petrolatum: 1 part by weight
Petrolatum: 17 parts by weight

Calculate the percentage strength for each ingredient. Must the percentages total 100%?

——————————————————————

A. 500 mg
B. 12.7 mL
C. 1.7 L
D. Boric acid: 10%
Liquid petrolatum: 5%
Petrolatum: 85%

Since all of the contributions in a w/w preparation are additive, the percentages must total 100%.

---

22. Calculating percentage strength in the apothecary system is much more complex than working in the metric system. Fortunately, apothecary prescriptions are seldom encountered. In the event that one should appear, the best procedure is to use the

metric system anyway. Since percent w/v is defined specifically in terms of grams and milliliters, changing to another set of units introduces unnecessary complexity. Start by converting the finished amount using the approximate equivalents:

$1 \mathfrak{Z} \approx 30$ g

$1 \, \mathrm{f} \mathfrak{Z} \approx 30$ mL

Then calculate the needed quantities in the usual way. Consider the prescription that follows:

℞

| Menthol | 1/2% |
| Alcohol qs ad | f ℥ ii |

The best procedure is to prepare 60 mL. The required amount of menthol is simply

60 mL $\times$ 0.005 g/mL = 0.3 g

℞

Iodine	2.5%
Potassium iodide	4.0%
Aqua dest qs ad	f ℥ i

Change the desired volume to metric units using the approximate equivalent and calculate the required number of grams of each ingredient.

- - - - - - - - - - - - - - - - - - - -

Iodine: 30 mL $\times$ 2.5 g/100 mL = 0.75 g
Potassium iodide: 30 mL $\times$ 4 g/100 mL = 1.2 g
Water: sufficient to make 30 mL

23. Imagine that a solution is prepared by dissolving 1 g of sodium chloride in sufficient water to make a total solution volume of 12 mL. As was explained in frame 14, the amount of water needed to make this solution cannot be calculated directly. This is because it is impossible to predict the amount of space occupied by the

dissolved sodium chloride. The density of pure, crystalline sodium chloride cannot be used to calculate the volume occupied by the salt in solution because the volume of a dissolved solute is almost always different from that of the pure material if it is a solid or gas. When liquids are combined into a solution, it sometimes happens that the volume of each liquid in the solution is the same as that in the pure state. This is most likely with liquids that are chemically similar. For example, 2.0 mL of decyl alcohol may be dissolved in 10.0 mL of octyl alcohol to produce 12.0 mL of solution. However, if 3.0 mL of ethanol are dissolved in 7.0 mL of water, the volume of the resulting solution is less than 10.0 mL. The volumes, in this case, are not additive. We can therefore state that, except for certain liquid mixtures, the volume of solution is not equal to the sum of the volumes of pure solute and pure solvent.

True or False:

A. The volume occupied by 1 g of hydrogen chloride in water solution is the same as that of 1 g of gaseous hydrogen chloride.
B. The volume occupied by 1 g of potassium bromide in water solution is the same as that of 1 g of solid potassium bromide.
C. The volume occupied by 1 g of methanol in water solution is the same as that of 1 g of pure liquid methanol.

––––––––––––––––––––––––––

All three statements are false.

24. If it should be necessary to determine the exact amount of solvent used in making a solution, we can make use of the fact that in contrast to volume, weight is always an additive property. That is,

weight of solute + weight of solvent = weight of solution

This equation is true for all solutions. Let us put it to use in the following example:
The specific gravity of a 25% w/v solution of sodium acetate in water is 1.113. How many milliliters of water should be used to prepare 40.0 mL of this solution?
According to the equation, we can find the *weight* of the solvent by subtracting the weight of the solute from the weight of the solution. Then, by using the density of the solvent (in this case, water) we can find the *volume* of solvent to use. Begin by calculating the weight of solute in 40 mL of solution.

40.0 mL × 0.25 g/mL = 10.0 g

25. Next, using the density of the solution, calculate the weight of 40.0 mL of solution.

    40.0 mL × 1.113 g/mL = 44.5 g

---

26. Now, determine the weight of solvent and then convert weight to volume by making use of its density.

    44.5 g − 10.0 g = 34.5 g

    $$34.5 \text{ g} \times \frac{1.00 \text{ mL}}{1.00 \text{ g}} = 34.5 \text{ mL}$$

---

27. Here is another problem.

    The formula for potassium iodide solution is:

    Potassium iodide (KI): 1000 g
    Purified water: a sufficient quantity to make 1000 mL

    How many milliliters of water will be needed to make 120 mL of solution? (The specific gravity of KI is 3.12; specific gravity of KI solution is 1.70.)

    _

    84 mL of water are required.

    If you ran into trouble, let us see if we can find what went wrong. Remember that the volume of solvent is found from its weight. Its weight is determined by subtracting the weight of solute from the weight of solution.
        I hope you did not try to make use of the density of KI. The volume of a material in solution is not the same as that of the pure substance. Go back to the problem. Find the number of grams of KI in 120 mL of the solution. Calculate the weight of the solution from its density. Determine the weight of water by difference and then the volume of water. The solution is shown in frame 28.

28. Since 1000 g of KI makes 1000 mL of solution, there will be 120 g of KI in 120 mL of solution. The weight of solution may be determined from its density:

120 mL × 1.70 g/mL = 204 g

204 g solution – 120 g KI = 84 g water

Since the density of water is 1.00 g per milliliter, 84 mL of water are required.

---

29. A manufacturer wishes to prepare 2 L of sodium acetrizoate solution, 30.0% w/v. The specific gravity of this solution is 1.195. How many milliliters of water will be required?

1790 mL

Solution:

Weight of the solution: 2000 mL × 1.95 g/mL = 2390 g

Weight of the sodium acetrizoate: 2000 mL × 0.300 = 600 g

Weight of the water: 2390 g – 600 g = 1790 g

Volume of the water: $1790 \text{ g} \times \dfrac{1 \text{ mL}}{1.00 \text{ g}} = 1790 \text{ mL water}$

---

30. How many milliliters of absolute alcohol must be used to make 240 mL of a 10% w/v solution of a drug? (Sp g absolute alcohol = 0.798; Sp g 10% solution of drug in absolute alcohol = 0.851.)

_ _

226 mL

Solution:

Weight of solution: 240 mL × 0.851 g/mL = 204 g

Weight of drug: 240 mL × 0.1 g/mL = 24 g

Weight of absolute alcohol: 204 g - 24 g = 180 g

Volume: $180 \text{ g} \times \dfrac{1 \text{ mL}}{0.798 \text{ g}} = 226 \text{ mL}$

---

31. The <u>USP</u> describes the solubility of drugs by stating the number of milliliters of solvent needed to dissolve 1 g of the drug. This type of information is useful if you want to be able to prepare a solution using the smallest amount of solvent possible. Such a solution is saturated with the solute.
    One gram of niacinamide dissolves in 1.5 mL of water. Calculate the volume of water needed to dissolve 12 g of niacinamide.

_ _

18 mL

Solution:

$$\frac{1 \text{ g}}{1.5 \text{ mL}} = \frac{12 \text{ g}}{j}$$

$j = 18 \text{ mL}$

---

32. How many grams of niacinamide would be contained in 100 g of a saturated solution of niacinamide in water? (Recall that 1 g dissolves in 1.5 mL of water.)

----

40 g

Solution:

When 1 g of the drug dissolves in 1.5 g of the solvent, 2.5 g of solution result. In other words, each 2.5 g of saturated solution contain 1 g of niacinamide.

$$\frac{1 \text{ g}}{2.5 \text{ g}} = \frac{j}{100 \text{ g}}$$

$$j = 40 \text{ g}$$

---

33. A gram of a drug dissolves in 12.0 mL of carbon tetrachloride (CCl_4). How many grams of the drug will be contained in 40.0 g of saturated solution? (Specific gravity of CCl_4 is 1.59.)

2.00 g

Solution:

g drug + g CCl_4 = g solution

In order to find the weight of solution that contains 1 g of the drug, we must determine the weight of 12.0 mL of CCl_4:

12.0 mL $\times$ 1.59 g/mL = 19.1 g

Therefore,

1 g drug + 19.1 g CCl_4 = 20.1 g solution

$$\frac{1 \text{ g drug}}{20.1 \text{ g solution}} = \frac{j}{40.0 \text{ g solution}}$$

$$j = 2.00 \text{ g of drug}$$

34. One gram of carbetapentane citrate dissolves in 6.5 mL of alcohol. What is the percentage strength of the solution w/w? (Sp g of alcohol is 0.814.)

_____

16% w/w

Solution:

$$6.5 \text{ mL} \times 0.814 \text{ g/mL} = 5.3 \text{ g}$$

Each gram of carbetapentane citrate dissolves in 5.3 g of alcohol yielding 6.3 g of solution.

$$\frac{1 \text{ g}}{6.3 \text{ g}} = 0.16 = 16\% \text{ w/w}$$

---

35. Using a percent is equivalent to stating the number of parts of solute in each 100 parts of solution. Parts per million (ppm) and parts per billion (ppb) are used to describe the concentration of very dilute solutions. ppm represents the number of parts of solute in 10^6 parts of solution. ppb describes the number of parts of solute in 10^9 parts of solution.

When ppm or ppb are used as a designation for concentration, some systems are w/w, some are v/v, and some are w/v. Concentration is always a ratio or fraction in w/w and v/v situations. w/v concentrations are always defined in terms of grams and milliliters. The same default rules are followed as for percentage systems.

If 10^6 mg (in other words, 1 kg) of a preparation contain 3 mg of a drug, the drug concentration is 3 ppm w/w. If 10^6 mL of a solution contain 22 mL of alcohol, the alcohol concentration is 22 ppm v/v. Any units may be used in describing w/w and v/v systems. However, with w/v situations, weight is in grams and volume is in milliliters. A 1.5 ppm w/v solution of a drug is one in which 10^6 mL of the solution contain 1.5 g of the drug.

A powder mixture contains 12 ppm of penicillin (as a contaminant). That is, each 10^6 g of powder contain 12 g of penicillin, or more generally, each 10^6 parts of the powder mixture contain 12 parts of penicillin.

The concentration of penicillin is therefore

$$\frac{12 \text{ parts}}{10^6 \text{ parts}} = 12 \times 10^{-6}$$

How many milligrams of penicillin are there in 5.6 kg of the powder mixture?

67.2 mg

Solution:

quantity of solute = concentration × quantity of preparation

$12 \times 10^{-6} \times 5.6 \text{ kg} = 67.2 \times 10^{-6} \text{ kg} = 67.2 \text{ mg}$

An alternative solution makes use of the definition directly. Since the concentration of penicillin is 12 ppm, each 10^6 mg of the mixture contain 12 mg of penicillin. The amount of penicillin in 5.6 kg (= 5.6×10^6 mg) of the mixture can be found by proportion.

$$\frac{12 \text{ mg}}{10^6 \text{ mg}} = \frac{j}{5.6 \times 10^6 \text{ mg}}$$

j = 67.2 mg penicillin

---

36. If 14 L of commercial ethyl alcohol are found to contain 0.010 mL of butanol, what is the concentration of butanol, in ppm?

0.71 ppm

Solution:

$$\text{concentration} = \frac{10 \times 10^{-3} \text{ mL}}{14 \times 10^3 \text{ mL}} = \frac{0.71}{10^6} = 0.71 \text{ ppm}$$

Or, by proportion,

$$\frac{0.010 \text{ mL}}{14 \times 10^3 \text{ mL}} = \frac{v}{10^6 \text{ mL}}$$

$v = 0.71$ mL of butanol. From the definition for ppm, the concentration is 0.71 ppm.

37. If the content of sodium fluoride in drinking water is 2 ppm, this means that in each 10^6 mL of this solution are contained 2 g of sodium fluoride. How many milligrams of sodium fluoride would be found in 15 L of the drinking water described above? (*Hint*: Sodium fluoride is a solid, so the concentration defaults to w/v and is expressed in terms of grams of solute and milliliters of solution.)

– –

30 mg

Solution:

2 ppm in this case is defined as 2 g in 10^6 mL

$$\frac{2 \text{ g}}{10^6 \text{ mL}} = \frac{j}{15 \times 10^3 \text{ mL}}$$

$j = 30 \times 10^{-3}$ g $= 30$ mg

38. The content of parathion (a solid) in a particular patient's bloodstream is 0.085 ppm. How many micrograms of parathion does her blood contain if her blood volume is 6.0 L?

----

510 µg

Solution:

$$\frac{0.085 \text{ g}}{10^6 \text{ mL}} = \frac{j}{6000 \text{ mL}}$$

$$j = 0.51 \times 10^{-3} \text{ g} = 510 \text{ µg}$$

---

39. A sample of a solution for injection is found to contain 1.4 ppm of lead chloride. How much of the solution will contain 50 µg of lead chloride?

----

36 mL

Solution:

1.4 ppm = 1.4 g in 10^6 mL; 50 µg = 50×10^{-6} g

$$\frac{1.4 \text{ g}}{10^6 \text{ mL}} = \frac{50 \times 10^{-6} \text{ g}}{j}$$

$$j = 36 \text{ mL}$$

---

40. The drinking water in a remote desert area in the Middle East contains 0.34 ppb of selenium. How many micrograms of selenium will be ingested by a camel whose water intake is 110 L?

37.4 µg

Solution:

$$\frac{0.34 \text{ g}}{10^9 \text{ mL}} \times (110 \times 10^3 \text{ mL}) = 37.4 \times 10^{-6} \text{ g} = 37.4 \text{ }\mu\text{g}$$

---

41. Here are some problems that review ppm and ppb calculations.

A. If 250 mL of water contain 0.275 mg of lead ion, what is the concentration of lead ion in ppm? In percent?

B. How many liters of solution can be prepared from 42.3 mg of an antioxidant if the final concentration of the antioxidant is supposed to be 12.0 ppm w/v?

C. If the methyl mercury content in a certain lake is 3.30 ppm, how many grams of methyl mercury would 250 L of lake water contain?

D. The asbestos level of a talc deposit is 0.79 ppb. How many micrograms of asbestos would be found in 10 g of this talc?

— —

A. 1.10 ppm; 1.10×10^{-4}%
B. 3.53 L
C. 0.825 g

D.   0.0079 µg

Solutions:

A. $\dfrac{0.275 \times 10^{-3} \text{ g}}{250 \text{ mL}} = \dfrac{j}{10^6 \text{ mL}}$

$j = 1.10$ g

That makes the concentration 1.10 ppm.

$\dfrac{0.275 \times 10^{-3} \text{ g}}{250 \text{ mL}} = \dfrac{j}{10^2 \text{ mL}}$

$j = 1.10 \times 10^{-4}$ g

The concentration is 1.10×10^{-4} g per 100 mL or $1.10 \times 10^{-4}\%$

B. $\dfrac{12 \text{ g}}{10^6 \text{ mL}} = \dfrac{42.3 \times 10^{-3} \text{ g}}{j}$

$j = 3.53$ L

C. $\dfrac{3.3 \text{ g}}{10^6 \text{ mL}} = \dfrac{j}{250 \times 10^3 \text{ mL}}$

$j = 0.825$ g

D. $\dfrac{0.79 \text{ g asbestos}}{10^9 \text{ g talc}} \times 10$ g talc $= 7.9 \times 10^{-9}$ g asbestos

= 0.0079 µg asbestos

---

42. If you need more practice with ppm problems, try these.

A.   What volume of solution can be prepared using 147 mg of sodium fluoride if the final concentration of sodium fluoride is to be 6.4 ppm?

B.   Express the concentration of alcohol in parts per million if 25.0 mL of blood of a reckless driver contained 9.50 µL of alcohol.

C. If 125 kg of rauwolfia (a plant drug) contain 8.5 mg of lead, what is the concentration of lead in parts per million?

D. The concentration of a preservative in a solution is 37.5 ppm, w/v. How many micrograms of the preservative will each teaspoonful contain?

E. The concentration of a pesticide in animal feed is 12.5 ppm. How many kilograms of animal feed would contain 0.65 mg of pesticide?

F. If the lead content in a patient's teeth is 15.0 ppm, how many micrograms of lead are bound there if the teeth weigh 15.0 g?

- - - - - - - - - - - - - - - - - - - -

A. 23 L
B. 380 ppm
C. 0.068 ppm
D. 188 µg
E. 0.052 kg
F. 225 µg

43. This is a good time to stop and review. Answer all of these
    questions before verifying your results.

A.   ℞

Salicylic acid	1.8 g
Benzoic acid	3.6 g
White ointment	54.6 g

What is the percentage strength of each of the three
components?

B. How many liters of a 0.2% solution in alcohol can be prepared using
   12.5 mL of spearmint oil?

C.   ℞

Glycerin	12%
Resorcinol	3.5%
Aq dest	50%
Alcohol qs ad	180.0 mL

How much glycerin and resorcinol (a solid) are needed for
this prescription?

D.   ℞

Hydrochloric acid, 10% w/v
Prepare 60.0 mL solution
Sig: 15 drops in water

How many grams of HCl does the patient receive in each
dose if the dropper dispensed with this medication delivers 32
drops/mL?

E. How many micrograms of a pesticide are present in 22.0 kg of a plant drug if the concentration of pesticide is 27.3 ppb?

F. ℞

Boric acid	2.5%
Epinephrine solution	2%
Aqua dest qs ad	15 mL

How much boric acid (a solid) and epinephrine solution are required?

G. How many liters of a 1.50% w/v potassium nitrate solution can be prepared from 22.0 g of potassium nitrate?

H. ℞

Vitamin C	100 mg
Iron	15 mg
d.t.d. caps No. LX	

How many grams of an iron choline citrate complex (containing 12% iron w/w) should be used in compounding this prescription?

I.   A pharmacist has to prepare 25.0 mL of a suspension containing 1/2% w/v of chloramphenicol. Instead of using pure chloramphenicol, she uses chloramphenicol palmitate, which contains 57.5% w/w chloramphenicol. How many milligrams of chloramphenicol palmitate should be used for this suspension?

J.   How many milliliters of water are required to prepare 75.0 mL of a 20% w/v solution of a salt? (Sp g of the salt solution = 1.12; sp g of the salt = 1.85; formula weight of the salt = 207.)

K.   Lanolin contains 72.5% w/w wool fat. The remainder is water. How many milliliters of water are there in 12.0 g of lanolin?

L.   Syrup is an 85% w/v solution of sucrose in water. It has a density of 1.313 g/mL. How many milliliters of water should be used to make 125 mL of syrup?

M.   If 1 g of a salt dissolves in 3.5 mL of water to form a saturated solution whose specific gravity is 1.10, how many grams will dissolve in 420 mL of water?

N. A gram of a salt dissolves in 4.90 mL of water to form a saturated solution whose specific gravity is 1.08. How many grams of the salt will be contained in 100 mL of the saturated solution?

O. ℞

       Elixir phenobarbital   120.0
    Sig: 1 teasp. tid

    Elixir phenobarbital contains 0.4% phenobarbital (w/v). How many milligrams of phenobarbital does the patient receive each day?

P. Phosphoric acid contains 86.5% w/w of H_3PO_4. How many grams of H_3PO_4 are contained in 55.0 mL of phosphoric acid? (Sp g of phosphoric acid = 1.71.)

Q. If 1 g of a drug dissolves in 2.50 mL of glycerin (sp g = 1.25), what is the percentage strength of the solution w/w?

R. An alkaloid extracted from a South American plant is found to be contaminated with DDT, 4 ppm. How many grams of the alkaloid will contain 20 mg of DDT?

S. If a source of drinking water contains 1.5 ppm of fluoride, how many micrograms of fluoride are present in one glass (240 mL) of water?

T. Express the concentration of alcohol in parts per million if 925 mL of fermentation broth contain 12.7 µL of alcohol.

_____

A. Salicylic acid: 3.00% w/w
    Benzoic acid: 6.00% w/w
    White ointment: 91.0% w/w
B. 6.25 L
C. Glycerin: 21.6 mL
    Resorcinol: 6.30 g
D. 0.047 g
E. 601 µg
F. Boric acid: 0.375 g
    Epinephrine solution: 0.3 mL
G. 1.47 L
H. 7.50 g
I. 217 mg
J. 69.0 mL
K. 3.30 mL
L. 57.8 mL
M. 120 g
N. 18.3 g
O. 60 mg
P. 81.4 g
Q. 24.2% w/w
R. 5000 g
S. 360 µg
T. 13.7 ppm

Solutions:

A. The formula is for a total of 60.0 g.

Salicylic acid: $\dfrac{1.8 \text{ g}}{60.0 \text{ g}} = 0.300 = 3\ 00\%$ w/w

Benzoic acid: $\dfrac{3.6 \text{ g}}{60.0 \text{ g}} = 0.0600 = 6.00\%$ w/w

White ointment: $\dfrac{54.6 \text{ g}}{60.0 \text{ g}} = 0.910 = 91.0\%$ w/w

B. $0.002 = \dfrac{12.5 \text{ mL oil}}{j}$

$j = 6250$ mL $= 6.25$ L solution

C.   Glycerin: 180 ml × 0.12 = 21.6 ml

Resorcinol: 180 mL × 0.035 g/mL = 6.3 g

D.   15 drops $\times \dfrac{1 \text{ mL}}{32 \text{ drops}} = 0.47$ mL

0.47 mL × 0.1 g/mL = 0.047 g

E. $\dfrac{27.3}{10^9} = \dfrac{j}{22 \text{ kg}}$

$j = 6.01 \times 10^{-7}$ kg = 601 µg

F.   Boric acid: 15 mL × 0.025 g/mL = 0.375 g

Epinephrine: 15 mL × 0.02 = 0.3 mL

G. 0.0150 g/mL $= \dfrac{22 \text{ g}}{j}$

$j = 1470$ mL = 1.47 L

H.   The total amount of iron needed is

15 mg/caps × 60 caps = 900 mg

$0.12 = \dfrac{900 \text{ mg}}{j}$

$j = 7500$ mg = 7.50 g

I.   25.0 mL × 0.005 g/mL = 0.125 g chloramphenicol

$$\frac{57.5 \text{ g}}{100 \text{ g}} = \frac{0.125 \text{ g}}{j}$$

$j = 0.217 \text{ g} = 217 \text{ mg}$

J.   Weight of solution: 75.0 mL × 1.12 g/mL = 84.0 g

Weight of salt: 75.0 mL × 0.2 g/mL = 15.0 g

Weight of solvent: 84.0 g − 15.0 g = 69.0 g = 69.0 mL

K.   The concentration of water must be 27.5% w/w

12.0 g × 0.275 = 3.30 g water = 3.30 mL

L.   125 mL × 0.85 g/mL = 106.25 g sucrose

125 mL × 1.313 g/mL = 164.1 g syrup

164.1 g − 106.3 g = 57.8 g water = 57.8 mL

M. $\dfrac{1 \text{ g}}{3.5 \text{ mL}} = \dfrac{j}{420 \text{ mL}}$

$j = 120 \text{ g}$

N.   1 g salt + 4.90 g H_2O = 5.90 g solution

$5.90 \text{ g} \times \dfrac{1 \text{ mL}}{1.08 \text{ g}} = 5.46 \text{ mL}$

$\dfrac{1 \text{ g salt}}{5.46 \text{ mL solution}} = \dfrac{j}{100 \text{ mL solution}}$

$j = 18.3 \text{ g}$

O.   The patient takes 15 mL per day:

15 mL × 0.004 g/mL = 0.060 g = 60 mg

P.   Since we know only the w/w concentration, only the weight of phosphoric acid allows us to calculate the H_3PO_4 content.

weight of phosphoric acid: 55 0 mL × 1.71 g/mL = 94.1 g

94.1 g × 0.865 = 81.4 g

Q.   We must know the weight of the drug in a definite weight of solution.

$$2.50 \text{ mL} \times 1.25 \text{ g/mL} = 3.13 \text{ g}$$

One gram of drug dissolves in 3.13 g of glycerin to make 4.12 g of solution.

$$\frac{1 \text{ g}}{4.13 \text{ g}} = 0.242 = 24.2\% \text{ w/w}$$

R. $$\frac{4 \text{ mg}}{10^6 \text{ mg}} = \frac{20 \text{ mg}}{j}$$

$$j = 5 \times 10^6 \text{ mg} = 5 \times 10^3 \text{ g}$$

S. $$\frac{1.5 \text{ g}}{10^6 \text{ mL}} = \frac{j}{240 \text{ mL}}$$

$$j = 360 \times 10^{-6} \text{ g} = 360 \text{ µg}$$

T. $$\frac{12.7 \text{ µL}}{925 \times 10^3 \text{ µL}} = \frac{j}{10^6 \text{ µL}}$$

$$j = 13.7 \text{ µL}$$

Therefore, the concentration is 13.7 ppm.

CHAPTER SEVEN

RATIO STRENGTH AND STOCK PREPARATIONS

Ratio strength is another way of representing concentration. In this convention, concentration is denoted in terms of the total amount of solution or mixture that contains one unit of solute. A *trituration* is a mixture containing a solid drug and an inert substance. Triturations and stock solutions provide a convenient means for handling a small quantity of potent drug.

Learning objectives: after completing this chapter the student should be able to

1. State the meaning of ratio strength expressions.
2. Calculate the quantity of drug in a given amount of a preparation whose concentration is expressed in terms of ratio strength.
3. Determine the amount of a preparation of given ratio strength that will contain a desired quantity of drug.
4. Determine the strength of a drug trituration to be prepared and the amount needed to supply a desired quantity of drug.
5. Calculate the quantity of a stock solution needed to deliver a desired quantity of drug.

---

1. As the name implies, ratio strength describes drug concentration in terms of a ratio. A 1:25 solution of cinnamon oil means that 1 mL of cinnamon oil is contained in each 25 mL of solution. Note that the second number in the ratio does not describe the quantity

---

of solvent or diluent, but rather the total quantity of the solution, which in this case includes cinnamon oil.

The very same default rules based on weighing of solids and volumetric measurement of liquids apply here. Thus, the cinnamon oil solution is assumed to be v/v since no other indication is given. Both liquids must have the same units. We can express this concentration as a percentage by first converting the ratio to a decimal value.

$$1:25 = 1 \text{ mL}:25 \text{ mL} = \frac{1 \text{ mL}}{25 \text{ mL}} = \frac{1}{25} = 0.04 \text{ v/v} = 4\% \text{ v/v}$$

What is the percentage strength of a 1:400 solution of an oil in alcohol?

0.25% v/v

Solution:

1:400 = 1 mL oil in 400 mL solution

Using proportion,

$$\frac{1 \text{ mL oil}}{400 \text{ mL solution}} = \frac{j}{100 \text{ mL}}$$

$j = 0.25$ mL oil

Since percent is defined as parts per 100, the strength of the solution is 0.25% v/v.

2. A 1:40 dilution of atropine in a solid mixture means that 1 g of atropine is contained in 40 g of the mixture. In systems of this type, the other solid material usually has no medicinal action. It is called a *diluent*. This type of solid mixture, containing only an active drug and diluent, is a *trituration*. Triturations provide a convenient means for handling materials used in very small quantities. The concentration of drug in the trituration is generally specified in terms of ratio strength.

The inert substance (or diluent) that is used most frequently in preparing triturations is lactose, otherwise known as milk sugar. Lactose has no drug action or ill effects and is pleasant tasting. In preparing a trituration, the drug and the diluent must be thoroughly mixed so that the resulting powder is completely uniform.

Notice that when both components are solids, they must have the same units. The concentration in this case is

$$1:40 = \frac{1 \text{ g}}{40 \text{ g}} = 0.025 \text{ w/w} = 2.5\% \text{ w/w}$$

What is the percentage strength of a 1:50 w/w mixture?

_____

2% w/w

Solution:

$$\frac{1}{50} = \frac{j}{100}$$

$j = 2$; 2 parts per 100 defines a 2% mixture.

3. A 1:1000 solution of thimerosal (a solid) means that 1 g of thimerosal is contained in each 1000 mL of the solution. As with percentage solutions, the ratio strength of w/v systems is defined in terms of grams (of solid) and milliliters (of liquid). The concentration is

$$\frac{1 \text{ g}}{1000 \text{ mL}} = 0.001 \text{ g/mL} = 0.1 \text{ g/100 mL or } 0.1\% \text{ w/v}$$

What is the percentage strength of a 1: 2000 w/v solution?

_ _

0.05% w/v

Solution:

$$\frac{1\ g}{2000\ mL} = \frac{j}{100\ mL}$$

j = 0.05 g; thus the concentration is 0.05%

---

4. Other expressions of concentration may be changed to ratio strength. The concentration is written as a fraction, reduced (so that the numerator has a value of "1"), and then converted to a ratio.

    If 3 mL of a liquid drug are dissolved in sufficient chloroform to make a total of 45 mL, the strength of the solution is

$$\frac{3\ mL}{45\ mL} = \frac{1}{15}$$

Thus the ratio strength is 1:15 v/v

    If 150 mg of strychnine sulfate are intimately mixed with 7.35 g of lactose, an inert substance, what is the ratio strength of strychnine sulfate in the mixture?

_ _

1:50 w/w

Solution:

    Total weight of the mixture:

    7.35 g + 0.15 g = 7.50 g

$$\frac{150\ mg}{7500\ mg} = \frac{1}{j}$$

j = 50; the ratio strength is 1:50

5. What is the ratio strength of a 0.01% w/v solution? (Remember that w/v systems are defined in terms of grams and milliliters.)

- -

1:10,000 w/v

Solution:

$$\frac{0.01\ g}{100\ mL} = \frac{1}{j}$$

j = 10,000; the strength is 1:10,000.

6. What is the ratio strength of a 0.5% solution of eucalyptus oil in mineral oil?

- -

1:200 v/v

Solution:

$$\frac{0.5\ mL\ oil}{100\ mL\ solution} = \frac{1\ mL\ oil}{j}$$

j = 200 mL of solution

The solution is therefore 1:200 v/v.

7. How many milligrams of mercury bichloride are needed to make 200 mL of a 1:500 w/v solution?

----

400 mg

Solution:

By definition, 500 mL of solution contain 1 g.

$$\frac{1 \text{ g}}{500 \text{ mL}} = \frac{j}{200 \text{ mL}}$$

$j = 0.4$ g $= 400$ mg

---

8. A pharmacist has 3.0 mL of an oil. How many milliliters of a 1:25 solution in alcohol can she prepare?

----

75 mL

Solution:

$$\frac{1}{25} = \frac{3.0 \text{ mL oil}}{j}$$

$j = 75$ mL solution

---

9. A 1:4 mixture containing codeine sulfate, with lactose as an inert diluent, is prepared. How many milligrams of lactose are present in 1.25 g of the mixture?

----

938 mg

Solution:

Since 4 parts of the mixture contain 1 part of drug, they must also contain 3 parts of lactose. The concentration of lactose is therefore

$$\frac{3 \text{ parts}}{4 \text{ parts}} = 0.75$$

$$0.75 \times 1.25 \text{ g} = 0.938 \text{ g} = 938 \text{ mg}$$

---

10. Here are some more ratio strength problems.

A. How many liters of a 1:1500 solution can be made by dissolving 4.80 g of cetylpyridinium chloride in water?

B. How many grams of quatricaine are needed to prepare 500 mL of a 1:800 w/v solution?

C. How many grams of lactose should be combined with 140 mg of a drug to make a 1:10 dilution?

D. The concentration of an antioxidant in an ointment is 1:250. How many milligrams of the antioxidant does each gram of the ointment contain?

E. What is the ratio strength of a drug if 260 mL of solution contain 0.65 µL of solute?

F. How many liters of a 1:500 solution of cinnamon oil in alcohol can be made from 27.5 mL of cinnamon oil?

G. What is the concentration (expressed as ratio strength) of phenylmercuric nitrate if 27.0 mL of the solution contain 45.0 mg of phenylmercuric nitrate?

H. The concentration of butyl alcohol in a whiskey is 0.04%. Express this concentration (1) in ppm; (2) in terms of ratio strength.

_ _

A. 7.2 L
B. 0.625 g
C. 1.26 g
D. 4 mg
E. 1:400,000
F. 13.8 L
G. 1:600
H. (1) 400 ppm; (2) 1:2500

11. Prescriptions and industrial formulas sometimes call for small quantities of drugs that are difficult or inconvenient to measure

using the usual instruments. If the final preparation is a solid, a stock solution may be used to deliver the drug, as in the following example.

A prescription for a skin lotion that uses alcohol as a base contains 0.63 g of menthol. The pharmacist has a 12% stock solution of menthol in alcohol. This solution can be used to provide the menthol needed for the lotion. Since, by definition, 100 mL of the stock solution contain 12 g of menthol, the volume containing 0.63 g would be found from

$$\frac{12.0 \text{ g}}{100 \text{ mL}} = \frac{0.63 \text{ g}}{j}$$

$$j = 5.25 \text{ mL}$$

5.25 mL of the menthol solution should be used for this prescription.

℞

Potassium permanganate	0.1 g
Aqua dest. q.s. ad	60.0 mL

How many milliliters of a 2.5% solution will yield the desired amount of potassium permanganate for this prescription?

_ _ _ _ _ _ _ _ _ _ _ _ _ _ _ _ _ _ _ _

4.00 mL

Solution:

$$\frac{2.5 \text{ g}}{100 \text{ mL}} = \frac{0.1 \text{ g}}{j}$$

$$j = 4.00 \text{ mL}$$

---

12. ℞

Boric acid	300 mg
Camphor water	7.0 mL
Aqua dest. q.s. ad	15.0 mL

How many milliliters of a 5% solution of boric acid in water should be used for this prescription?

_ _

6.00 mL

Solution:

$$\frac{5 \text{ g}}{100 \text{ mL}} = \frac{0.3 \text{ g}}{j}$$

$j = 6.00$ mL

---

13. ℞

Cocaine HCl	90.0 mg
Boric acid solution	3.0 mL
Aqua pur. q.s. ad	7.5 mL

How many milliliters of a 1:40 solution of cocaine HCl in water should be used for this prescription?

_ _ _ _ _ _ _ _ _ _ _ _ _ _ _ _ _ _ _ _

3.60 mL

Solution:

$$\frac{1 \text{ g}}{40 \text{ mL}} = \frac{0.09 \text{ g}}{j}$$

$j = 3.60$ mL

---

14. Try your hand at the calculations that follow.

A. ℞

Menthol   300 mg
Mineral oil q.s. ad   30.0 mL

How many milliliters of a 15% stock solution of menthol in mineral oil should be used to fill this prescription?

B. A pharmacist needs 1.95 grams of a salt for a prescription. How many milliliters of a 32.5% solution of the salt are needed?

A.   2.0 mL
B.   6.0 mL

Solutions:

A. $\dfrac{15\ g}{100\ mL} = \dfrac{0.3\ g}{j}$

$j = 2.0\ mL$

B. $\dfrac{32.5\ g}{100\ mL} = \dfrac{1.95\ g}{j}$

$j = 6.0\ mL$

15. The trituration is also a stock preparation, one in which a solid drug is intimately dispersed with a solid, inert diluent. Since both components are solids, they are measured by weight so that triturations are always w/w systems.

What is the concentration, in ratio strength, of a trituration made by combining 120 mg of atropine sulfate and 3.48 g of lactose?

- - - - - - - - - - - - - - - - - - - -

1:30

Solution:

Remember that the strength of a trituration is expressed as a ratio of active ingredient to total weight In this case, the total weight is

$$0.120 \text{ g} + 3.48 \text{ g} = 3.60 \text{ g}$$

$$\frac{0.120 \text{ g}}{3.60 \text{ g}} = \frac{1}{j}$$

$$j = 30$$

The concentration is 1:30

---

16. ℞

Strychnine sulfate	45 mg
Belladonna extract	360 mg
Sucrose	36.0 g

Ft. chart; Div. in #XXXVI

How many grams of a 1:80 trituration of strychnine sulfate should be used for this prescription?

- - - - - - - - - - - - - - - - - - - -

3.60 g

Solution:

We wish to know the quantity of trituration that contains 45 mg of strychnine sulfate. One approach is to use proportion:

$$1:80 = \frac{1}{80} = \frac{45 \text{ mg}}{j}$$

$$j = 3600 \text{ mg} = 3.60 \text{ g}$$

Another possibility that leads to the same result is to rearrange the concentration equation:

$$\text{concentration} = \frac{\text{amount of solute}}{\text{amount of preparation}}$$

to

$$\text{amount of preparation} = \frac{\text{amount of solute}}{\text{concentration}}$$

In the example,

$$\frac{45 \text{ mg}}{\dfrac{1}{80}} = 3600 \text{ mg} = 3.60 \text{ g}$$

---

17. How many grams of a 1:25 trituration of saccharin sodium are needed to make 30 mL of a solution containing 2 mg of saccharin sodium in each milliliter?

1.50 g

Solution:

Total saccharin sodium needed:

$$2 \text{ mg/mL} \times 30 \text{ mL} = 60 \text{ mg}$$

$$\frac{60 \text{ mg}}{\dfrac{1}{25}} = 1500 \text{ mg} = 1.50 \text{ g}$$

18. ℞

Atropine sulfate	0.4 mg
Sodium bicarbonate	0.4 g
Pepsin	0.2 g
Lactose	q.s.

d.t.d. chart No. 30

How many milligrams of a 1:40 trituration of atropine sulfate (in lactose) should be weighed for this prescription?

––––––––––––––––––––––––––

480 mg

Solution:

Total quantity of atropine sulfate needed:

0.4 mg/chart × 30 chart = 12 mg

$$\frac{12 \text{ mg}}{\frac{1}{40}} = 480 \text{ mg}$$

19. It is necessary to prepare a 1:15 trituration of emetine sulfate in sucrose. How much sucrose should be combined with 200 mg of emetine sulfate to make this trituration?

––––––––––––––––––––––––––

2800 mg

Solution:

$$\frac{200 \text{ mg}}{\frac{1}{15}} = 3000 \text{ mg total trituration}$$

$$3000 \text{ mg} - 200 \text{ mg} = 2800 \text{ mg}$$

20. A pharmacist wishes to prepare a 1:12 trituration of codeine phosphate, using lactose as the diluent. How many grams of lactose should be used to make the trituration if the pharmacist employs the smallest quantity of codeine phosphate that can be weighed on a prescription balance with acceptable accuracy?

_____

1.32 g

Solution:

The minimum weighable quantity on the prescription balance is 120 mg.

$$\frac{120 \text{ mg}}{\frac{1}{12}} = 1440 \text{ mg}$$

$$1440 \text{ mg} - 120 \text{ mg} = 1320 \text{ mg} = 1.32 \text{ g lactose}$$

21. Try these problems for review and practice:

A. A prescription calls for 16 mg of atropine. How many grams of a 1:30 dilution of atropine in lactose will supply the needed amount of atropine?

B. What is the ratio strength of a trituration made by combining 0.25 g of a drug with 2.75 g of lactose?

C. A pharmacist needs 5 mg of a drug. How many milligrams of a 1:30 dilution of the drug should she use?

_ _

A. 0.48 g
B. 1:12
C. 150 mg

22. When quantities smaller than 120 mg are prescribed, they cannot be weighed directly on a prescription balance. Some other means for measuring the weight of a drug accurately must be found. Sometimes the drug will be available in tablets. It is then possible to calculate the number of tablets that will supply the required amount of drug.

Another approach to the measurement of small quantities involves the use of stock solutions and triturations. In these preparations, the diluent expands the weight (or volume) of the system, allowing convenient and accurate measurement. A stock preparation allows us to obtain the necessary amount of the drug without compromising accuracy.

Thirty-five milligrams of morphine sulfate are needed for a prescription. It is not possible to weigh less than 120 mg with acceptable accuracy on a prescription balance, but the difficulty can be circumvented by using a trituration as the source of the drug. If a 1:10 trituration is available, how many milligrams of the trituration should be used?

----

350 mg

$$\frac{35 \text{ mg}}{\frac{1}{10}} = 350 \text{ mg of trituration}$$

The pharmacist should use 350 mg of the trituration. This quantity can be weighed with acceptable accuracy using a prescription balance.

---

23. A prescription requires 35 mg of morphine sulfate. How should the pharmacist proceed?
     The question posed here is similar to that in frame 22 except that no trituration is available. The pharmacist must prepare one himself. A suitable quantity of morphine sulfate (at least 120 mg) must be combined with an inert substance like lactose. A portion of the trituration will then be used to obtain 35 mg of morphine sulfate.

A. A 1:10 trituration may be prepared. Then (as we saw in frame 22) 350 mg of trituration will be used for the prescription.

B. A 1:7 trituration may be prepared. The amount required would be

$$\frac{35 \text{ mg}}{\frac{1}{7}} = 245 \text{ mg trituration}$$

245 mg of a 1:7 trituration would be used. This is also acceptable since 245 mg exceeds the minimum weighable quantity for a prescription balance.

C. A 1:3 trituration may be prepared. The amount required would be

$$\frac{35 \text{ mg}}{\frac{1}{3}} = 105 \text{ mg trituration}$$

105 mg of a 1:3 trituration are needed. Unfortunately, this is not an acceptable approach because 105 mg is not a weighable quantity. It is below the minimum weighable amount for the instrument.

Referring to the calculations above, does the quantity of trituration needed to deliver a fixed amount of drug have to be reduced, increased, or remain unchanged as the concentration of the trituration is increased?

—————————————————————————

Reduced (1:3 is a higher concentration than 1:7)

---

24. If the concentration of the trituration is made too high, the amount of trituration that contains the desired quantity of drug will be less than 120 mg and will therefore not be a weighable quantity.

  To obtain the maximum permissible strength of the trituration, find the smallest whole number by which the required drug amount should be multiplied to give at least 120 mg. The trituration is the reciprocal of this number.

  For example, let us say that 40 mg of a drug has to be weighed. 40 mg must be multiplied by 3 to equal 120 mg. A 1:3 trituration should be prepared. The amount of trituration necessary to supply 40 mg of the drug is 120 mg:

$$\frac{40 \text{ mg}}{\frac{1}{3}} = 120 \text{ mg}$$

  As a second example, assume that 22 mg of a drug has to be weighed. The smallest whole number by which 22 mg must be multiplied to equal or just exceed 120 mg is 6. Therefore, a 1:6 trituration should be prepared. 132 mg of the trituration are required for the prescription:

$$\frac{22 \text{ mg}}{\frac{1}{6}} = 132 \text{ mg}$$

  For the following situations, determine the trituration of maximum strength that could be used to supply the necessary amount of drug

A.   55 mg of drug are needed.
B.   14 mg of drug are needed.
C.   80 mg of drug are needed.

A.   1:3
B.   1:9
C.   1:2

25. Now let us consider a practical problem: A pharmacist has to weigh 25 mg of a drug for a prescription. This quantity is less than 120 mg and cannot be weighed directly on a prescription balance. We must resort to using a trituration. Our calculation consists of three steps:

(1) Determine the strength of the trituration.

(2) Determine the quantities needed to make the trituration.

(3) Determine the amount of trituration that contains the desired quantity of drug.

We work these out as follows:

(1) By inspection, 25 mg must be multiplied by 5 to give a product of at least 120 mg. Use a 1:5 trituration.

(2) To make the 1:5 trituration, weigh 120 mg of the drug and mix intimately with 480 mg of lactose (or another inert material, perhaps one included in the prescription).

(3) Calculate the amount of trituration needed.

$$\frac{25 \text{ mg}}{\frac{1}{5}} = 125 \text{ mg}$$

125 mg of the trituration should be used for the prescription. If lactose is not part of the prescription formula, it is permissible for the pharmacist to add it to the formula because lactose is inert and will do no harm.

Note that a concentration weaker than 1:5 could have been used to solve the problem. Use of weaker dilutions will be just as accurate. But the use of large quantities may lead to practical difficulties. If the drug is being incorporated into a powder mass that will be divided into capsules, the use of excessively dilute triturations may involve such large quantities of material that the capsules will be too large to swallow. Review the procedure for weighing quantities less than 120 mg. Then try this problem:

A pharmacist has a prescription for 6 capsules, each capsule to contain 8 mg of phenobarbital. How should the phenobarbital be weighed?

_____

The total needed is

8 mg/caps × 6 caps = 48 mg

A trituration of phenobarbital must be prepared.

(1) Use a 1:3 trituration.

(2) To make the 1:3 trituration, combine 120 mg of phenobarbital with 240 mg of diluent.

(3) $\dfrac{48 \text{ mg}}{\frac{1}{3}}$ = 144 mg

Weigh 144 mg of the trituration. It will contain 48 mg of phenobarbital.

---

26. ℞

Aspirin	600 mg
Caffeine	30 mg
Codeine sulfate	12 mg
Lactose qs	

d.t.d. capsules #6

How can the codeine sulfate be weighed?

_____

The total needed is

12 mg/caps × 6 caps = 72 mg

We must make up a trituration. Lactose may be used as the diluent.

(1) Use a 1:2 trituration.

(2) Prepare a 1:2 trituration by mixing 120 mg of codeine sulfate with 120 mg of lactose.

(3) $\dfrac{72 \text{ mg}}{\frac{1}{2}}$ = 144 mg

The trituration will contain 72 mg of codeine sulfate and 72 mg of lactose.

---

27. Do all of the following review problems before checking your answers:

A. How many milligrams of Zephiran chloride are required to make 1 L of a 1:750 solution in water?

B. A solution of potassium permanganate (1:2500) is used as a fungicide on a turtle's shell. If the shell is of such size as to require 1.2 mL of the solution for complete coverage, how many micrograms of potassium permanganate will be put on the shell?

C. How much kaolin should be used to prepare 2.00 g of a 1:30 dilution of hyoscine in kaolin? Both substances are solids.

D. What is the ratio strength of a solution in which 18.0 mg of solute is dissolved in sufficient water to make a total of 450 mL?

E. How many liters of a 1:800 solution can be made by dissolving 0.60 g of a drug in water?

F. The concentration of a sweetener in a solution is 1:400 w/v. How many milligrams of the sweetener does each teaspoonful contain?

G. How many milliliters of a 4% stock solution of silver nitrate contain 150 mg of silver nitrate?

H. How many grams of lactose should be added to 120 mg of strychnine sulfate to make a 1:20 trituration?

I. How many milligrams of a 1:25 trituration of atropine should be used to prepare 40 capsules, each containing 0.4 mg of atropine?

J. A prescription for capsules calls for 18 mg of a drug. Calculate the maximum concentration of a trituration of simple ratio that may be used as a source of the drug.

K. R︎

       Hyoscine hydrobromide   0.001 g
       Benadryl hydrochloride   0.025 g
   d.t.d. caps No. 12

    How would you weigh the hyoscine hydrobromide for this prescription?

- -

A. 1330 mg
B. 480 µg
C. 1.93 g
D. 1:25,000
E. 0.48 L
F. 12.5 mg
G. 3.75 mL
H. 2.28 g
I. 400 mg
J. 1:7
K. Combine 120 mg of drug with 1.08 g of lactose and mix thoroughly. Use 120 mg of the mixture. (Other answers that give the same amount of drug in the final step are also correct.)

Solutions:

A. $\dfrac{1\,g}{750\ mL} = \dfrac{j}{1000\ mL}$

    $j = 1.33\ g = 1330\ mg$

B. $\dfrac{1 \text{ g}}{2500 \text{ mL}} = \dfrac{j}{1.2 \text{ mL}}$

$j = 4.8 \times 10^{-4} \text{ g} = 4.8 \times 10^{2} \text{ µg}$

C. The concentration of kaolin in the mixture is 29/30 w/w:

$\dfrac{29}{30} = \dfrac{j}{2.00}$

$j = 1.93 \text{ g}$

D. $\dfrac{0.018 \text{ g}}{450 \text{ mL}} = \dfrac{1 \text{ g}}{j}$

$j = 25{,}000 \text{ mL}$

concentration = 1:25,000

E. $\dfrac{1 \text{ g}}{800 \text{ mL}} = \dfrac{0.60 \text{ g}}{j}$

$j = 480 \text{ mL} = 0.48 \text{ L}$

F. $\dfrac{1 \text{ g}}{400 \text{ mL}} = \dfrac{j}{5 \text{ mL}}$

$j = 0.0125 \text{ g} = 12.5 \text{ mg}$

G. $\dfrac{0.150 \text{ g}}{4 \text{ g}/100 \text{ mL}} = 3.75 \text{ mL}$

H. $\dfrac{120 \text{ mg}}{\dfrac{1}{20}} = 2400 \text{ mg trituration}$

2400 mg − 120 mg = 2280 mg = 2.28 g

I. 0.4 mg/caps × 40 caps = 16 mg

$\dfrac{16 \text{ mg}}{\dfrac{1}{25}} = 400 \text{ mg}$

J. 18 mg × 7 = 126 mg

1:7 may be used.

K.   1 mg/cap × 12 cap = 12 mg

12 mg × 10 = 120 mg

Make a 1:10 trituration by combining 120 mg of drug with 1080 mg of a diluent such as lactose.

$$\frac{12 \text{ mg}}{\frac{1}{10}} = 120 \text{ mg}$$

CHAPTER EIGHT

DILUTION AND CONCENTRATION

In previous chapters we have dealt with preparations in which the drug content is expressed as a concentration. It may be necessary to dilute concentrated systems prior to use. Sometimes the dilution is performed by the pharmacist and sometimes by the patient. On occasion, the strength of active ingredient may have to be raised. Sometimes, components of varying strength must be blended to arrive at a product whose strength satisfies a required standard. All of these problems may be handled by essentially the same calculation technique.

Learning objectives: after completing this chapter the student should be able to

1. Calculate the amount of a preparation to be diluted to yield a preparation of lower strength.
2. Determine the quantity of a preparation to be combined with another preparation containing the same active ingredient to yield a preparation of intermediate strength.
3. Determine the concentration of a mixture prepared by combining preparations of different concentration.
4. Calculate the amount of active ingredient needed to prepare a concentrate that is to be diluted by the patient prior to use.

1. An important equation for us in this chapter is

    quantity of solute = concentration × quantity of preparation

Calculate the amount of drug present in 300 mL of a 4.0% w/v solution of that drug.

_____

0.040 g/mL × 300 mL = 12 g

2. Using the same equation, calculate the amount of alcohol present in 35 mL of a 60% solution of alcohol in water.

_____

0.60 × 35 mL = 21 mL

3. Using the same equation, calculate the amount of calamine in 13 g of a 10% w/w calamine ointment.

_____

(0.10) (13 g) = 1.3 g

4. Calculate the number of milligrams of potassium permanganate in 90 mL of a 1:500 w/v potassium permanganate solution.

‒ ‒

180 mg

Solution:

$$90 \text{ mL} \times \frac{1 \text{ g}}{500 \text{ mL}} = 0.18 \text{ g} = 180 \text{ mg}$$

5. Try these problems.

A. How many milliliters of solute are there in
    (1) 350 mL of 5% v/v solution?
    (2) 4.20 L of a 1:2000 v/v solution?

B. How many grams of solute are there in
    (1) 220 g of a 1:40 w/w solution?
    (2) 170 mL of a 15.0% w/v solution?

C. How many milligrams of drug are there in
    (1) 25.0 mL of a 3.25% w/v solution?
    (2) 900 g of a 1:150 w/w mixture?

‒ ‒

A. (1) 17.5 mL
    (2) 2.1 mL
B. (1) 5.5 g
    (2) 25.5 g
C. (1) 813 mg
    (2) 6000 mg

6. It is sometimes necessary for the pharmacist to dilute a stock preparation to make a product of lower strength. Here is an example:

℞

Ichthammol ointment 8% w/w   90.0 g
Ft. ung.

The pharmacist has some 20% w/w ichthammol ointment. He wishes to dilute it with petrolatum, an inert semisolid that contains no drug of any kind, to the proper strength. The quantity of the 20% ointment and of petrolatum to be mixed must be determined.

The key to solving problems of this type is the realization that the amount of an ingredient in the finished product must be equal to the contributions of the components of the formula. In terms of our example, we know that the ichthammol in our final product, the 8% ointment, must be the sum of the ichthammol contributed by the 20% ichthammol ointment and by the petrolatum. We may therefore write

g ichthammol from 20% ointment + g ichthammol from petrolatum = g ichthammol in 8% ointment

To conserve space, I am going to rewrite this equation, which is called a *mass balance equation*, using a bit of shorthand. The preparation that contains the ingredient will be written in parentheses, and "ichthammol" will be abbreviated as "ich."

g ich (20% oint) + g ich (petrolatum) = g ich (8% oint)

Of course, there is no ichthammol in petrolatum, so our equation becomes

g ich (20% oint) = g ich (8% oint)

Recall that

g ich = (concentration) (quantity of preparation)

Let j equal the quantity of 20% ointment to be used:

g ich (20% oint) = 0.20 j

g ich (8% oint) = (0.08) (90.0 g) = 7.2 g

Substituting these quantities in our mass balance equation yields

(0.20) j = 7.20 g

$$j = \frac{7.20 \text{ g}}{0.20} = 36 \text{ g}$$

Use 36 g of the 20% ichthammol ointment; the amount of petrolatum needed is 90 g − 36 g = 54 g.

To solve problems involving dilution or concentration:

(1) Write the mass balance equation.
(2) Substitute in the mass balance equation.
(3) Solve the resulting algebraic expression.

---

7. We wish to dilute an ointment containing 14% sulfur with petrolatum to make 60 g of an ointment containing 10% sulfur. Write a mass balance equation that shows where the sulfur in the finished product (the 10% ointment) comes from.

    _

    g S (14% oint) = g S (10% oint). (Petrolatum contains no sulfur.)

---

8. Calculate the amount of sulfur in the 10% ointment using the equation

    quantity of solute = concentration × quantity of preparation

    _

    g S (10% oint) = (0.100) (60 g) = 6 g

---

9. Let j equal the quantity of 14% ointment to be used. Calculate the number of grams of sulfur in the 14% ointment.

    _

    g S (14% oint) = 0.14 j

---

10. Substitute in the mass balance equation and solve.

—————————————————————

$0.14\,j = 6$ g

$j = 42.9$ g

Use 42.9 g of the 14% sulfur ointment. (The amount of petrolatum is 60.0 g − 42.9 g = 17.1 g.)

---

11. It is necessary to prepare 180 mL of a 1:200 solution of potassium permanganate ($KMnO_4$). What quantity of a 5% stock solution of $KMnO_4$ should be diluted with water?
    Fill in the blank in the mass balance equation:

    _____ = g $KMnO_4$ (1:200 sol)

    ———————————————————————

    g $KMnO_4$ (5% sol)

---

12. Let j equal the number of milliliters of 5% $KMnO_4$ solution to be diluted. Fill in the blanks:

A. g $KMnO_4$ (5% sol) = _____

B. g $KMnO_4$ (1:200 sol) = _____

    ———————————————————————

    A. (0.05 g/mL) j
    B. $\dfrac{1\ \text{g}}{200\ \text{mL}} \times 180\ \text{mL} = 0.9$ g

---

13. Now, substitute in the mass balance equation and solve.

    (0.05 g/mL) j = 0.9 g

    $j = \dfrac{0.9\ \text{g}}{0.05\ \text{g/mL}} = 18$ mL

Use 18 mL of the 5% solution.
    How many milliliters of a 10% w/v merthiolate solution should be diluted with water to make 440 mL of a 0.25% w/v merthiolate solution?

----

11 mL

Solution:

Let j equal the milliliters of 10% merthiolate solution:

g merth (10%) = g merth (0.25%)

$(0.10 \text{ g/mL}) j = (440 \text{ mL}) (0.0025 \text{ g/mL}) = 1.1 \text{ g}$

$j = 11 \text{ mL}$

---

14. How many milliliters of water must be added to 180 mL of 36% w/v acetic acid solution in order to make up a solution of 10% w/v strength? (Assume that no shrinkage or expansion of volume occurs on mixing.)

----

468 mL

Solution:

Let j equal the quantity of water to be added. The volume of the 10% solution will then be 180 mL $+ j$.

g acetic acid (36% sol) = g acetic acid (10% sol)

$(0.36 \text{ g/mL}) (180 \text{ mL}) = (0.1 \text{ g/mL}) (180 \text{ mL} + j)$

$64.8 \text{ g} = 18.0 \text{ g} + (0.1 \text{ g/mL}) j$

$$j = \frac{64.8 \text{ g} - 18.0 \text{ g}}{0.1 \text{ g/mL}} = 468 \text{ mL}$$

15. How many milliliters of Zephiran concentrate (17% w/v of Zephiran) are required to prepare 2 L of a 1:1500 solution of Zephiran?

7.84 mL

Solution:

Let j equal the milliliters of Zephiran concentrate needed:

g Zephiran (17% sol) = g Zephiran (1:1500 sol)

(0.17 g/mL) j = (1/1500 g/mL) (2000 mL)

j = 7.84 mL

16. If 12.5 g of a 10% zinc oxide ointment are diluted with 17.5 g of white petrolatum, what is the percentage strength of the resulting product?

4.17%

Solution:

Let j equal the concentration of the diluted ointment:

g zinc oxide (10% oint) = g zinc oxide (dil oint)

(0.1) (12.5 g) = (j) (30.0 g)

$j = \dfrac{(0.1)\,(12.5\text{ g})}{30.0\text{ g}} = 0.0417 = 4.17\%$

17. How much 22% v/v solution of glycerin in water can be made by diluting 90 mL of an 80% v/v glycerin solution with water?

_ _

327 mL

Solution:

Let j equal the volume of diluted solution:

$$(0.8)\,(90\ \text{mL}) = 0.22\,j$$

$$j = \frac{72\ \text{mL}}{0.22} = 327\ \text{mL}$$

18. How many grams of petrolatum should be added to 15% sulfur ointment to make 120 g of a 6.5% sulfur ointment?

_ _

68 g

Solution:

Let j equal the amount of petrolatum to add:

$$(0.15)\,(120\ \text{g} - j) = (0.065)\,(120\ \text{g})$$

$$18\ \text{g} - 0.15\,j = 7.8\ \text{g}$$

$$j = \frac{7.8\ \text{g} - 18\ \text{g}}{-0.15} = 68\ \text{g}$$

19. Hydrochloric acid USP is a 36% w/w solution of HCl in water with a specific gravity of 1.18. How many milliliters should be used to prepare 200 mL of a 5% w/v solution of HCl?

——————————————————————

23.6 mL

(If you ran into trouble, go to frame 20 for a hint. If you were successful, go to frame 21.)

20. The mass balance equation is

    g HCl (36% w/w sol) = g HCl (5% w/v sol)

We cannot set j equal to volume of 36% w/w HCl solution and multiply 0.36 by j to get the amount of HCl. j is a volume; 0.36 refers to concentration on a weight basis. The two quantities are just not compatible. However, it is possible to calculate the weight of the 36% solution and then convert that to volume using its density. Try the problem again. If you still have difficulty, consult the solution.

——————————————————————

Solution:

Let j equal the weight of hydrochloric acid needed:

$$0.36\, j = (0.05 \text{ g/mL}) (200 \text{ mL})$$

$$j = \frac{(0.05 \text{ g/mL}) (200 \text{ mL})}{0.36} = 27.8 \text{ g}$$

$$27.8 \text{ g} \times \frac{1 \text{ mL}}{1.18 \text{ g}} = 23.6 \text{ mL}$$

Use 23.5 mL of hydrochloric acid USP.

---

21. A pharmacist wishes to prepare 150 mL of ammonia (NH_3) solution, 10% w/v. How many milliliters of strong ammonia solution (28.5% w/w) should be used? (Sp g of strong ammonia solution is 0.900.)

- -

58.4 mL

Solution:

Let j equal the weight of 28.5% solution to be used:

g NH_3 (28.5% w/w sol) = g NH_3 (10% w/v sol)

$0.285\,j = (0.1 \text{ g/mL}) (150 \text{ mL})$

$j = 52.6 \text{ g}$

$52.6 \text{ g} \times \dfrac{1 \text{ mL}}{0.900 \text{ g}} = 58.4 \text{ mL}$

---

22. A crude drug is required to contain 0.28% w/w of an alkaloid, the active compound. How many kilograms of a batch of crude drug containing 0.30% w/w alkaloid must be combined with 500 g of crude drug containing 0.20% w/w alkaloid in order that the resulting mixture will meet the required standard? (*Hint*: Use the same procedure as for previous problems in this chapter; write the mass balance equation and then substitute in it.)

- -

2.0 kg

(If you were able to solve this problem, go to frame 26. If you need help, go to frame 23.

23. The mass balance equation is

g alkaloid (0.20%) + g alkaloid (0.30%) = g alkaloid (0.28%)

Let j equal the quantity of 0.30% crude drug required. Can you go on from here? Try the problem again. If you still have trouble, go to frame 24.

24. Let j equal the quantity of 0.30% crude drug necessary:

g alkaloid (0.20%) = (500 g) (0.0020)

g alkaloid (0.30%) = 0.0030 j

g alkaloid (0.28%) = (500 g + j) (0.0028)

Now complete the solution.

_____

25. The solution is as follows:

g alkaloid (0.20%) + g alkaloid (0.30%) = g alkaloid (0.28%)

(500 g) (0.0020) + 0.0030 j = (500 g + j) (0.0028)

1.0 g + 0.0030 j = 1.4 g + 0.0028 j

j = 2000 g = 2.0 kg

26. How many milliliters of a syrup containing 85.0% w/v sucrose should be mixed with 115 mL of a syrup containing 60.0% w/v sucrose to prepare a syrup containing 76.0% w/v sucrose? (Assume that there is no expansion or shrinkage of volume when the two liquids are mixed.)

_ _ _ _ _ _ _ _ _ _ _ _ _ _ _ _ _ _ _ _

204 mL

Solution:

Let j equal the volume of 85% sucrose:

g sucrose (85%) + g sucrose (60%) = g sucrose (76%)

(0.85 g/mL) (j) + (0.60 g/mL) (115 mL)

$\quad$ = (0.76 g/mL) (115 mL + j)

0.85 j + 69 g = 87.4 g + 0.76 j

j = 204 mL

---

27. How many milliliters of 0.5% sodium sulfate solution should be mixed with 5.0% sodium sulfate solution to make 1 L of a 2% solution?

_ _ _ _ _ _ _ _ _ _ _ _ _ _ _ _ _ _ _ _

667 mL of 0.5% solution

Solution:

Let j equal the milliliters of 0.5% solution. Since the finished product measures 1000 mL,

(1000 mL − j) = volume of the 5% solution needed

g sod sulf (0.5%) + g sod sulf (5%) = g sod sulf (2%)

(j) (0.005 g/mL) + (1000 mL − j) (0.05 g/mL)

$\quad$ = (1000 mL × 0.02 g/mL)

(j) (0.005 g/mL) + 50 g − (j) (0.05 g/mL) = 20 g

j = 667 mL

---

28. ℞

Belladonna tincture	20.0 mL (67% C_2H_5OH)
Elixir phenobarbital	70.0 mL (15% C_2H_5OH)
Alcohol USP qs	
Syrup tolu qs ad	180.0 mL

How much alcohol USP (95% C_2H_5OH) should be used in this prescription in order that the concentration of ethanol (C_2H_5OH) in the finished product be 20% v/v?

- - - - - - - - - - - - - - - - - -

12.7 mL

Solution:

Let j equal the milliliters of alcohol USP needed:

mL eth (67%) + mL eth (15%) + mL eth (95%)

= mL eth (product)

(20.0 mL) (0.67) + (70.0 mL) (0.15) + 0.95 j = (180) (0.20)

13.4 mL + 10.5 mL + 0.95 j = 36.0 mL

j = 12.7 mL

---

29. If 300 g of an ointment containing 4% (w/w) sulfur is combined with 220 g of a 10% (w/w) sulfur ointment, what is the strength of the mixture that results?

6.54% w/w

Solution:

Let j equal the strength of finished product:

g S (4% oint) + g S (10% oint) = g S (mixture)

(300 g) (0.04) + (220 g) (0.1) = (520 g) (j)

j = 0.0654 = 6.54%

---

30. A pharmacist combines 140 mL of a 0.90% sodium chloride solution with 250 mL of 3.4% sodium chloride solution. Assuming no expansion or contraction in volume, calculate the percentage strength of the mixture.

2.5%

Solution:

Let j equal the concentration of the mixture:

g NaCl (0.90%) + g NaCl (3.4%) = g NaCl (mixture)

(140 mL) (0.0090 g/mL) + (250 mL) (0.034 g/mL)

= (390 mL) (j)

j = 0.025 g/mL = 2.5%

---

31. ℞

Phenobarbital elixir	40.0 mL
High alcoholic elixir	40.0 mL
Syrup qs ad	120.0 mL

What is the ethanol percentage in the finished product? Phenobarbital elixir contains 15% C_2H_5OH; high alcoholic elixir contains 78% C_2H_5OH. Syrup contains no ethanol.

31% v/v

Solution:

Let j equal the concentration of the finished product:

mL C_2H_5OH (pheno elix) + mL C_2H_5OH (h.a. elix)

= mL C_2H_5OH (product)

(40.0 mL) (0.15) + (40.0 mL) (0.78) = 120 mL (j)

$j = 0.31 = 31\%$ v/v

---

32. Here are some problems that review the material covered in this chapter so far.

A. If 4.0 mL of a 5.0% benzethonium chloride solution are diluted with water to 500 mL, what will the ratio strength of the resulting solution be?

B. How much 14% sodium solution should be diluted with water to make 350 mL of 6% sodium acetate solution?

C. How much lanolin (an inert ointment base) should be added to 300 g of cortisone ointment, 3%, to make an ointment containing cortisone, 1:250?

D. A pharmacist needs 60 mL of diluted acetic acid (a 6% w/v solution of $C_2H_4O_2$ in water) for a prescription. The pharmacist has only acetic acid USP on hand. This is a 36% w/w solution of $C_2H_4O_2$ in water with a specific gravity of 1.045.

How many milliliters of acetic acid USP should the pharmacist use?

E. How much pure zinc oxide should be mixed with a 10.0% zinc oxide ointment to make 3.75 kg of a 12.0% zinc oxide ointment?

F. Three samples of a plant have the following potencies:

Sample 1 (220 g) contains 2.40% alkaloids
Sample 2 (50.0 g) contains 1.97% alkaloids
Sample 3 (450 g) contains 3.85% alkaloids

If the three samples are combined, what is the alkaloid content, expressed as a percent, of the mixture?

G. What is the percentage of benzalkonium chloride in a solution made by mixing 350 mL of a 1:100 benzalkonium chloride solution with 250 mL of a 1:300 benzalkonium chloride solution?

H. ℞

    Phenobarbital elixir (15% C_2H_5OH)   30 mL
    High-alcoholic elixir (78% C_2H_5OH) qs
    Elixir terpin hydrate (42% C_2H_5OH)   45 mL
    Syrup qs ad   120 mL

    How many milliliters of high-alcoholic elixir should be used to make the C_2H_5OH content of the final solution 35%?

————————————————————

A. 1:2500
B. 150 mL
C. 1950 g
D. 9.6 mL
E. 83.3 g
F. 3.27%
G. 0.722%
H. 23.8 mL

---

33. Occasionally, the pharmacist is asked to dispense a stock solution that will be diluted by the patient prior to use.
    A phenylmercuric nitrate concentrate has a concentration of 4% w/v. What is the final concentration, in terms of ratio strength, in a solution made by diluting 1 teaspoonful of the concentrate to 200 mL?

————————————————————

1:1000

Solution:

Let j equal the concentration of diluted solution:

$$(5 \text{ mL}) (0.04 \text{ g/mL}) = (200 \text{ mL}) (j)$$

$$j = 0.001 \text{ g/mL} = 1{:}1000$$

---

34. How many milliliters must 1 tablespoonful of the concentrate be diluted to in order to yield a 1:1500 solution of phenylmercuric nitrate?

_ _

900 mL

Solution:

Let j equal the volume of diluted solution:

$$(0.04 \text{ g/mL}) (15 \text{ mL}) = \frac{1 \text{ g}}{1500 \text{ mL}} j$$

$$j = 900 \text{ mL}$$

---

35. ℞

      Potassium permanganate solution   60.0

Make of such strength that 1 teaspoonful diluted to a liter will yield a 1:10,000 solution.

Calculate the number of grams of potassium permanganate ($KMnO_4$) needed to make the solution.

Two approaches to this problem are possible. One way is to calculate the concentration of the prescription solution and then find the amount of $KMnO_4$ needed to make the solution.

The second method which is somewhat easier, is to calculate the number of grams of $KMnO_4$ in the diluted solution. This quantity must also be contained in 1 teaspoonful of the stock solution dispensed to the patient. If you can get this far, you can calculate the amount of $KMnO_4$ required for 60.0 mL of the stock solution.

_____

1.20 g

Solution:

g $KMnO_4$ in 1 teasp concentrate = g $KMnO_4$ in diluted sol

$$= \frac{1 \text{ g}}{10^4 \text{ mL}} \times 1000 \text{ mL} = 0.1 \text{ g}$$

Therefore, each teaspoonful of the stock solution contains 0.1 g of $KMnO_4$. We must prepare a total of 60.0 mL, or 12 teaspoonfuls.

0.100 g/teaspoonful × 12 teaspoonfuls = 1.20 g

36. ℞
    Silver nitrate qs
Ft sol, 30.0 mL
Each teaspoonful diluted to a pint yields a 1:5000 solution.

How many grams of silver nitrate ($AgNO_3$) should be used to make this solution? (Since the measuring devices in the average household are not as accurate as those available to the pharmacist, a pint may be approximated by 500 mL in the calculation.)

_____

0.6 g

Solution:

The amount of $AgNO_3$ in the diluted solution is

$$\frac{1\ g}{5000\ mL} \times 500\ mL = 0.1\ g$$

This is also the content of each teaspoonful of the concentrate:

0.1 g/teaspoonful × 6 teaspoonfuls = 0.6 g

---

37. If you would like additional practice, here are some more problems dealing with situations in which the patient must make the dilution.

A. ℞

Benzethonium chloride solution   60 mL
One teaspoonful diluted to 500 mL yields a 1:1500 solution.

How many grams of benzethonium chloride are needed?

B. A phenylmercuric acetate concentrate is to be prepared. One tablespoonful of the concentrate is diluted to 500 mL with water to yield a 1:2000 solution of phenylmercuric acetate. What must be the percentage concentration of phenylmercuric acetate in the concentrate?

C. ℞

Phenylmercuric nitrate solution   180 mL
One teaspoonful diluted to a pint yields a 1:2500 solution.

How many grams of phenylmercuric nitrate should be used for the solution? (Use 1 pt = 500 mL, since the patient will make the dilution.)

A.   4.00 g
B.   1.67%
C.   6.91 g

---

38. Do all of the problems before verifying your answers.

A.   ℞

Benzalkonium chloride qs
Aqua dest. qs ad   180.0 mL
One tablespoonful diluted to a liter yields a 1:750 solution.

How many grams of benzalkonium chloride should be used to make this solution?

B.   How many milliliters of 95% alcohol should be diluted with water to make 65.0 mL of 40% alcohol?

C.   A lotion is made by mixing 250 mL of witch hazel (14% C_2H_5OH), 1 L of diluted alcohol (49% C_2H_5OH), and sufficient water to make 2 L. What is the percentage strength of C_2H_5OH in the lotion?

D.   How much 20% sulfathiazole ointment should be added to 200 g of 6% sulfathiazole ointment to make an ointment of 10% strength?

E. Belladonna tincture is required to contain 30 mg of alkaloids in each 100 mL of the tincture. If 250 mL of the tincture is prepared and the assay shows the alkaloids content to be 0.035%, how much solvent should be used to dilute the tincture so that it meets the standard requirement?

F. How much 4.5% sodium acetate solution can be made from 32 mL of a 12% sodium acetate solution?

G. If 142 g of petrolatum are mixed with 25 g of 0.20% mercury bichloride ointment, what will the final concentration of mercury bichloride be?

H. How many milliliters of a 15% solution of sodium chloride should be used to make 1 L of a 0.9% solution of sodium chloride?

I. How many grams of pure coal tar should be added to 36.0 g of 4.0% coal tar ointment to make a 10% coal tar ointment?

J. We need 90 mL of phosphoric acid solution, 10% w/v. How many milliliters of phosphoric acid USP (85% w/w; sp g = 1.71) should be used?

K. ℞

$$Phenobarbital\ elixir\ (15\%\ C_2H_5OH)\quad 20.0\ mL$$

Alcohol USP (95% C_2H_5OH)
Syrup tolu (no C_2H_5OH) qs ad   90.0 mL

How much alcohol USP should be used in this prescription to bring the C_2H_5OH content of the final preparation to 20%?

_____

A. 16.0 g
B. 27.4 mL
C. 26.3%
D. 80 g
E. 42 mL
F. 85 mL
G. 0.030%
H. 60 mL
I. 2.4 g
J. 6.2 mL
K. 15.8 mL

Solutions:

A. benzethonium chloride = 1/750 g/mL × 1000 mL = 1.33 g

Each tablespoonful of the stock solution contains 1.33 g:

1.33 g/tablespoonful × 12 tablespoonfuls = 16.0 g

B. Let j equal the volume of alcohol, 95%:

mL ethanol (95%) = mL ethanol (40%)

$0.95 \, j = (65.0 \text{ mL}) (0.4)$

$j = 27.4 \text{ mL}$

C. Let j equal the strength of the lotion:

mL eth (w. h.) + mL eth (dil alc) = mL eth (lotion)

$(250 \text{ mL}) (0.14) + (1000 \text{ mL}) (0.49) = (2000 \text{ mL}) \, j$

$$j = \frac{35 \text{ mL} + 490 \text{ mL}}{2000 \text{ mL}} = 0.263 = 26.3\%$$

D. Let j equal the grams of 20% ointment:

g sulfa (20% oint) + g sulfa (6% oint) = g sulfa (10% oint)

$j \, (0.20) + (200 \text{ g}) (0.06) = (200 \text{ g} + j) (0.10)$

$j = 80 \text{ g}$

E. Let j equal the milliliters of solvent:

g alkaloids (0.035% tr) = g alkaloids (0.030% tr)

$(250 \text{ mL}) (0.00035 \text{ g/mL}) = (250 \text{ mL} + j) (0.00030 \text{ g/mL})$

$0.0875 \text{ g} = 0.075 \text{ g} + (0.00030 \text{ g/mL}) \, (j)$

$j = 42 \text{ mL}$

F. Let j equal the milliliters of 4.5% solution:

g sod acetate (4.5%) = g sod acetate (12%)

$(0.045 \text{ g/mL}) \, j = (0.12 \text{ g/mL}) (32 \text{ mL})$

$j = 85 \text{ mL}$

G. Let j equal the final concentration:

g $HgCl_2$ (0.20%) = g $HgCl_2$ (final product)

$(25 \text{ g}) (0.002) = (167 \text{ g}) \, j$

$j = 0.00030 = 0.030\%$

H. Let j equal the milliliters of 15% solution:

g NaCl (15%) = g NaCl (0.9%)

$(0.15 \text{ g/mL}) \, j = (0.009 \text{ g/mL}) (1000 \text{ mL})$

$j = 60 \text{ mL}$

I.   Let j equal the grams of pure coal tar:

g coal tar + g coal tar (4% oint) = g coal tar (10% oint)

$j + (36.0 \text{ g}) (0.04) = (36.0 + j) (0.10)$

$j + 1.44 \text{ g} = 3.60 \text{ g} + 0.1 \, j$

$0.9 \, j = 2.16 \text{ g}$

$j = 2.4 \text{ g}$

J.   Let j equal the grams of phosphoric acid USP to be used:

g H_3PO_4 (concentrate) = g H_3PO_4 (10% solution)

$0.85 \, j = (90 \text{ mL}) (0.10 \text{ g/mL})$

$j = 10.6 \text{ g}$

$10.6 \text{ g} \times \dfrac{1 \text{ mL}}{1.71 \text{ g}} = 6.20 \text{ mL}$

K.   Let j equal the milliliters of alcohol USP to be added:

mL eth (alc USP) + mL eth (pheno elix) = mL eth (product)

$0.95 \, j + (0.15) (20 \text{ mL}) = (0.20) (90 \text{ mL})$

$j = 15.8 \text{ mL}$

CHAPTER NINE

MILLLIEQUIVALENTS

Certain ions are of critical importance in maintaining normal body function. When an essential ion is lost through disease, it must be replaced. Salts are usually used as sources of needed ions for this type of therapy.

Sometimes the necessary amount of the salt will be stated on the prescription. Alternatively, the physician will prescribe some quantity of the needed ion, and the pharmacist will be asked to calculate how much salt will contain that quantity.

Although quantities may be denoted in the usual units of weight, chemical units, particularly milliequivalents, are more commonly used. Your knowledge of elementary inorganic chemistry will be very helpful.

Learning objectives: after completing this chapter the student should be able to

1. Express quantities in terms of moles, millimoles, equivalents and milliequivalents.
2. Calculate the amount of an electrolyte that will yield a desired quantity of one of its component ions.
3. Determine the amount of an electrolyte that will supply a desired concentration or quantity of a component ion expressed as millimoles.
4. Determine the number of millimoles per unit volume from a knowledge of the quantity of electrolyte used.

1. Some properties of the elements in which we are most interested are listed in Table 9–1.

    Table 9–1. Atomic Weight and Valence of Selected Elements

Element	Atomic Weight	Usual Valence
calcium	40.0	+2
carbon	12.0	
chlorine	35.5	−1
fluorine	19.0	−1
hydrogen	1.0	+1
magnesium	24.3	+2
oxygen	16.0	−2
potassium	39.1	+1
sodium	23.0	+1
sulfur	32.1	

    Try these problems as a review. Recall that the number of moles of a reactant or product is indicated by the coefficient which precedes that species in the chemical equation.

A. Write the chemical equation for the dissociation of calcium nitrate.
B. How many moles (mol) result from the dissociation of 1 mol of sodium sulfate?
C. How many moles of magnesium chloride are necessary to yield 1 mol of magnesium ion?
D. How many moles of magnesium chloride are necessary to yield 1 mol of chloride ion?

- -

A. $Ca(NO_3)_2 = Ca^{2+} + 2NO_3^-$
B. 3 mol
C. 1 mol
D. 1/2 mol

Solutions:

A.   Shown above.

B. $Na_2SO_4 = 2Na^+ + SO_4^{2-}$

Each mole of sodium sulfate yields 2 mol of sodium and 1 mol of sulfate.

C. $MgCl_2 = Mg^{2+} + 2Cl^-$

Each mole of magnesium chloride yields 1 mol of magnesium ion and 2 mol of chloride.

D.   See solution C.

---

2.   One mole (or gram molecular weight) of a substance is defined as the formula weight for that substance, expressed in grams.

A.   How many grams of sodium chloride are equivalent to 1 mol?
B.   How many moles are equivalent to 45.0 g of potassium carbonate?

- -

A.   58.5 g
B.   0.326 mol

Solutions:

A.   Na: 23.0
     Cl: 35.5
     Total: 58.5

     1 mol = 58.5 g

B.   K: 78.2
     C: 12.0
     3 O: 48.0
                138.2

     1 mol of potassium carbonate = 138.2 g

     $$45.0 \text{ g} \times \frac{1 \text{ mol}}{138.2 \text{ g}} = 0.326 \text{ mol}$$

3. The chemical equation relates quantities in terms of moles. By converting moles to grams, relationships in weight may be obtained. In the case of anhydrous sodium carbonate, for example,

$$Na_2CO_3 = 2Na^+ + CO_3^{2-}$$

Each mole of sodium carbonate contains 2 mol of sodium. The molecular weight of sodium carbonate is 106. Therefore, 106 g of sodium carbonate contain 46.0 g of sodium.

How many grams of anhydrous sodium carbonate contain 350 mg of sodium?

_ _

0.807 g

Solution:

$$\frac{106.0 \text{ g}}{46.0 \text{ g}} = \frac{j}{0.350 \text{ g}}$$

$$j = 0.807 \text{ g}$$

4. How many grams of sodium carbonate decahydrate $(Na_2CO_3 \cdot 10H_2O)$ contain 350 mg of sodium?

_ _

2.18 g

Solution:

$$Na_2CO_3 \cdot 10H_2O = 2Na^+ + CO_3^{2-} + 10H_2O$$

The molecular weight of the salt is 286:

$$\frac{286 \text{ g}}{46.0 \text{ g}} = \frac{j}{0.350 \text{ g}}$$

$$j = 2.18 \text{ g}$$

---

5. Calculate the percentage of calcium in calcium carbonate.

40.0%

Solution:

Calcium has an atomic weight of 40.0.
$CaCO_3$ has a molecular weight of 100.0.

$$\frac{40.0}{100.0} = 40.0\%$$

---

6. It is recommended that drinking water contain 1 ppm of fluoride
    to strengthen bones and teeth. How many grams of sodium
    fluoride should be added to 10,000 L of drinking water containing
    0.25 ppm of fluoride ion to provide the optimum concentration?
    (*Hint*: first calculate the amount of fluoride ion to add; then
    determine the amount of NaF that will contain the needed
    amount of fluoride.)

----

17 g

Solution:

We may write the following mass balance equation:

g F⁻ (original water) + g F⁻ (added) = g F⁻ (treated water)

Let j equal the quantity of fluoride to be added. (The increase in volume due to the added NaF is negligible.) Substituting in the mass balance equation gives

$$(0.25 \times 10^{-6} \text{ g/mL}) (10^7 \text{ mL}) + j = (1 \times 10^{-6} \text{ g/mL}) (10^7 \text{ mL})$$

$$j = 10 \text{ g} - 2.5 \text{ g} = 7.5 \text{ g}$$

We have calculated the amount of fluoride to add.

$$NaF = Na^+ + F^-$$

g atomic wt of $F^- = 19.0$

g molecular wt of $NaF = 42.0$

In 42.0 g of sodium fluoride there are 19.0 g of fluoride.

$$\frac{19.0 \text{ g}}{42.0 \text{ g}} = \frac{7.5 \text{ g}}{j}$$

$$j = 17 \text{ g}$$

---

7. A manufacturer has prepared sodium fluoride solution, 0.44% W/V. If the dropper supplied with the package delivers 1.0 mL of this solution in 30 drops, how many drops will contain 1.0 mg of fluoride?

- -

15 drops

Solution:

$$NaF = Na^+ + F^-$$

42.0 g of sodium fluoride contain 19.0 g of fluoride.

$$\frac{19.0 \text{ g}}{42.0 \text{ g}} = \frac{1.0 \text{ mg}}{j}$$

$j = 2.2$ mg

We must determine the number of drops of the solution that will contain 2.2 mg of sodium fluoride (which is equivalent to 1.0 mg of F^-). First, calculate the number of milliliters:

0.44% W/V = 0.0044 g/mL = 4.4 mg/mL

$$\frac{2.2 \text{ mg}}{4.4 \text{ mg/mL}} = 0.50 \text{ mL of NaF solution}$$

0.50 mL × 30 drops/mL = 15 drops

---

8. A mole, or gram molecular weight, is the molecular weight expressed in grams. A millimole (mmol) is the molecular weight expressed in milligrams. It is a measure of quantity, not concentration.

A. How many milligrams of sodium chloride represent 0.5 mmol?

B. How many millimoles are there in 3.2 g of calcium fluoride?

— — — — — — — — — — — — — — — — — —

A. 29.3 mg
B. 41 mmol

Solutions:

A. molecular wt of NaCl = 58.5

    58.5 mg NaCl = 1 mmol

0.5 mmol = 29.3 mg

B.   molecular wt of CaF_2 = 78.0

78.0 mg CaF_2 = 1 mmol

$$3200 \text{ mg} \times \frac{1 \text{ mmol}}{78.0 \text{ mg}} = 41 \text{ mmol}$$

---

9.   A prescription calls for 24 mmol of potassium chloride. How many grams of KCl are required?

_____

1.79 g

Solution:

molecular wt of KCl = 74.6

74.6 mg = 1 mmol

$$24 \text{ mmol} \times \frac{74.6 \text{ mg}}{1 \text{ mmol}} = 1790 \text{ mg} = 1.79 \text{ g}$$

---

10.   How many millimoles are there in 1.50 g of Epsom salts $(MgSO_4 \cdot 7H_2O)$?

_____

6.09 mmol

Solution:

molecular wt of $MgSO_4 \cdot 7H_2O$ = 246.4

$$246.4 \text{ mg} = 1 \text{ mmol}$$

$$1500 \text{ mg} \times \frac{1 \text{ mmol}}{246.4 \text{ mg}} = 6.09 \text{ mmol}$$

---

11. How many grams of sodium chloride should be used to prepare this solution?

   ℞

   NaCl solution   90.0 mL

   Each 5 mL contains 0.6 mmol of Na^+.

— —

0.632 g

Solution:

   0.6 mmol/teaspoonful × 18 teaspoonfuls = 10.8 mmol Na^+

   $NaCl = Na^+ + Cl^-$

From this equation we see that each mole of sodium chloride yields 1 mol of Na^+. Therefore, 10.8 mmol of Na^+ will be supplied by 10.8 mmol of NaCl. Thus

   molecular wt NaCl = 58.5

   58.5 mg NaCl = 1 mmol

   10.8 mmol × 58.5 mg/mmol = 632 mg = 0.632 g

---

12. How many grams of anhydrous sodium sulfate should be used to prepare the following prescription?

   ℞

   Sodium sulfate solution   60.0 mL

   Each milliliter contains 0.1 mmol of Na^+.

0.426 g

Solution:

$0.1 \text{ mmol/mL} \times 60 \text{ mL} = 6 \text{ mmol Na}^+$

$Na_2SO_4 = 2Na^+ + SO_4^{2-}$

Each mole of sodium sulfate yields 2 mol of Na^+.

$$\frac{1 \text{ mol } Na_2SO_4}{2 \text{ mol } Na^+} = \frac{j}{6 \text{ mmol } Na^+}$$

$j = 3 \text{ mmol } Na_2SO_4$ needed

molecular wt $Na_2SO_4 = 142.1$

$3 \text{ mmol} \times 142.1 \text{ mg/mmol} = 426 \text{ mg} = 0.426 \text{ g}$

---

13. Try these review problems:

A. How many grams of calcium fluoride should be used to prepare 300 kg of a toothpaste containing 0.015% of fluoride ion?

B. How many millimoles of sulfate ion are there in 60.0 mL of a 3.50% sodium sulfate solution?

C. A pharmacist is to prepare 150 mL of a solution of magnesium sulfate containing 1 mmole of magnesium ion per milliliter. How many grams of magnesium sulfate should be used?

D. How many grams of calcium fluoride should be used to make
    35.0 mL of a solution that is to contain 9.00 ppm of fluoride ion?

E. How many millimoles of chloride ion are there in 30.0 mL of a
    2.00% calcium chloride solution?

- -

A. 92.4 g
B. 14.8 mmol
C. 18.1 g
D. 6.47 × 10⁻⁴ g
E. 10.8 mmol

Solutions:

A. 300×10^3 g $\times 0.00015 = 45$ g F⁻

Each 78.0 g of CaF_2 contains 38.0 g of F⁻.

$$\frac{38.0}{78.0} = \frac{45 \text{ g}}{j}$$

$j = 92.4$ g

B. 60 mL × 0.035 g/mL = 2.1 g Na_2SO_4

Each mole of Na_2SO_4 contains 1 mol of SO_4^{2-}.

142.1 mg Na_2SO_4 contain 1 mmol SO_4^{2-}

$$2.1 \text{ g} \times \frac{1 \text{ mmol}}{142.1 \text{ mg}} = 14.8 \text{ mmol}$$

C. $150 \text{ mL} \times 1 \text{ mmol/mL} = 150 \text{ mmol}$

$120.4 \text{ mg } MgSO_4 = 1 \text{ mmol Mg}$

$150 \text{ mmol} \times 120.4 \text{ mg/mmol} = 18{,}100 \text{ mg} = 18.1 \text{ g}$

D. $\dfrac{9 \text{ g}}{10^6 \text{ mL}} = \dfrac{j}{35 \text{ mL}}$

$j = 3.15 \times 10^{-4} \text{ g } F^-$

$\dfrac{38.0}{78.0} = \dfrac{3.15 \times 10^{-4} \text{ g}}{k}$

$k = 6.47 \times 10^{-4} \text{ g } CaF_2$

E. $30 \text{ mL} \times 0.02 \text{ g/mL} = 0.6 \text{ g } CaCl_2$

$CaCl_2 = Ca^{2+} + 2Cl^-$

$111 \text{ mg } CaCl_2 = 2 \text{ mmol } Cl^-$

$600 \text{ mg} \times \dfrac{2 \text{ mmol}}{111 \text{ mg}} = 10.8 \text{ mmol}$

---

14. The mole and millimole are convenient units because they are directly related to the chemical equation. Another unit often used in connection with electrolytes is the equivalent. Whenever a chemical change occurs, 1 equivalent of a positively charged ion combines with 1 equivalent of a negatively charged ion. When a salt dissociates, the same number of equivalents of positive and of negative ions are produced.

   The number of equivalents is found by multiplying the number of moles by the absolute value of the valence.

A.   How many equivalents of K^+ are produced by the dissociation of 1 mol of potassium carbonate?

B.   How many equivalents of $CO_3{}^{2-}$?

A.   2
B.   2

Solutions:

A. $K_2CO_3 = 2K^+ + CO_3^{2-}$

Thus 2 mol of K^+ are produced.

moles × valence = equivalents

2 × 1 = 2 equivalents of K^+

B.   Only 1 mol of carbonate is produced.

moles × valence = equivalents

1 × 2 = 2 equivalents of CO_3^{2-}

Notice that the equivalents of cation and anion are equal in number.

---

15. The equivalent is often too large a unit for calculation. The milliequivalent (mEq), 1/1000 of an equivalent, is widely used. The number of milliequivalents is found by multiplying the number of millimoles by the absolute value of the valence.
    How many milliequivalents of fluoride ion are contained in 0.35 g of potassium fluoride?

_ _

6.02 mEq

Solution:

$KF = K^+ + F^-$

1 mEq F^- = 1 mmol F^- = 1 mmol KF = 58.1 mg

$$350 \text{ mg KF} \times \frac{1 \text{ mEq F}^-}{58.1 \text{ mg KF}} = 6.02 \text{ mEq F}^-$$

16. If 10 mEq of Cl^- are desired, how many milligrams of $CaCl_2$ should be used?

----

555 mg

Solution:

$$CaCl_2 = Ca^{2+} + 2\ Cl^-$$

1 mmol $CaCl_2$ = 2 mmol Cl^- = 2 mEq Cl^-= 111 mg $CaCl_2$

$$10\ \text{mEq Cl}^- \times \frac{111\ \text{mg CaCl}_2}{2\ \text{mEq Cl}^-} = 555\ \text{mg CaCl}_2$$

---

17. How many milliequivalents of magnesium ion are there in each teaspoonful of a 2% solution of magnesium chloride?

2.10 mEq

Solution:

$$(5\ mL \times 0.02\ g/mL) = 0.1\ g\ MgCl_2$$

$$MgCl_2 = Mg^{2+} + 2\ Cl^-$$

1 mmol $MgCl_2$ = 95.3 mg = 1 mmol Mg^{2+} = 2 mEq Mg^{2+}

$$100\ \text{mg MgCl}_2 \times \frac{2\ \text{mEq Mg}^{2+}}{95.3\ \text{mg MgCl}_2} = 2.10\ \text{mEq Mg}^{2+}$$

18. How many milliliters of a 10% potassium chloride solution must the patient take to obtain 5.0 mEq of K^+?

3.73 mL

Solution:

$KCl = K^+ + Cl^-$

1 mEq K^+ = 1 mmol K^+ = 1 mmol KCl = 74.6 mg

5.0 mEq $K^+ \times \dfrac{74.6 \text{ mg KCl}}{1 \text{ mEq } K^+} = 373$ mg KCl

$\dfrac{0.373 \text{ g}}{0.10 \text{ g/mL}} = 3.73$ mL

19. How many grams of $CaCl_2 \cdot 2H_2O$ should be used to prepare 180 mL of a calcium chloride solution containing 2.5 mEq of calcium ion in each teaspoonful?

6.62 g

Solution:

2.5 mEq/teaspoonful × 36 teaspoonfuls = 90 mEq needed

$CaCl_2 \cdot 2H_2O = Ca^{2+} + 2Cl^- + 2H_2O$

$$1 \text{ mmol } Ca^{2+} = 2 \text{ mEq } Ca^{2+} = 1 \text{ mmol } CaCl_2 \cdot 2H_2O$$

$$= 147.0 \text{ mg } CaCl_2 \cdot 2H_2O$$

$$90 \text{ mEq } Ca^{2+} \times \frac{147.0 \text{ mg } CaCl_2 \cdot 2H_2O}{2 \text{ mEq } Ca^{2+}} = 6620 \text{ mg}$$

$$= 6.62 \text{ g } CaCl_2 \cdot 2H_2O$$

---

20. How many grams of magnesium chloride should be used to prepare 60 mL of a solution intended to contain 1.5 mEq of magnesium ion per milliliter?

_ _

4.29 g

Solution:

$$60 \text{ mL} \times 1.5 \text{ mEq/mL} = 90 \text{ mEq}$$

$$MgCl_2 = Mg^{2+} + 2Cl^-$$

$$1 \text{ mmol } Mg^{2+} = 2 \text{ mEq } Mg^{2+} = 1 \text{ mmol } MgCl_2 = 95.3 \text{ mg}$$

$$90 \text{ mEq} \times \frac{95.3 \text{ mg}}{2 \text{ mEq}} = 4290 \text{ mg} = 4.29 \text{ g}$$

---

21. If you would like more practice, try your hand at these problems:

A. If 2.86 g of magnesium chloride are used to prepare 120 mL of a solution, how many milliequivalents of magnesium ion will each teaspoon contain?

B. How many grams of potassium chloride should be used to prepare
    90 mL of a solution containing 0.8 mEq of K^+/mL?

C. ℞

    Solution calcium chloride 5%   180 mL
    Sig: 1 teaspoonful tid

    How many milliequivalents of chloride ion does the patient
    receive each day?

D. ℞

    Potassium sulfate to yield 1.0 mEq of K^+
    Aqua qs ad   5.0 mL
    d.t.d. #24
    Sig: 5.0 mL b.i.d.

    How many grams of potassium sulfate should be used for this
    prescription?

E. If city water contains 2.5 ppm of NaF, calculate the number of
    milliequivalents of fluoride ingested by a person who drinks 1.5 L
    of water.

F. A solution is prepared by dissolving 8.42 g of sodium chloride in
    sufficient water to make 180 mL of solution. In how many
    milliliters will 8 mEq of sodium ion be contained?

A. 2.50 mEq
B. 5.37 g
C. 13.5 mEq
D. 2.09 g
E. 0.089 mEq
F. 10.1 mL

---

22. Do all of these problems before verifying your answers.

A. How many grams of potassium carbonate will contain the same quantity of potassium as 3.50 g of potassium chloride?

B. How many millimoles of chloride ion are present in 1 teaspoonful of a 10% solution of magnesium chloride?

C. If the fluoride content of a dentifrice is to be 0.25%, how many grams of sodium fluoride should be used per kilogram of toothpaste?

D. How many milliliters of a 6.0% solution of magnesium sulfate contain 5.0 mmol of magnesium ion?

E. How many milliequivalents of chloride ion does each tablespoonful
    of a 3.5% potassium chloride solution contain?

F. How many milliliters of a 5% solution of $MgCl_2$ contain 20 mEq
    of Mg^{2+}?

G. How many grams of K_2SO_4 should be used to prepare 240 mL of
    a potassium sulfate solution to contain 1 mEq K^+/mL?

H. How many milliequivalents of chloride ion are contained in each
    milliliter of a 0.9% sodium chloride solution?

I. ℞

        Calcium chloride solution, 7.5 mEq Ca^{2+}/teaspoonful
    Ft 120 mL

        How many grams of calcium chloride should be used to
    prepare this prescription?

A. 3.25 g
B. 10.5 mmol
C. 5.53 g
D. 10 mL
E. 7.04 mEq
F. 19.1 mL
G. 20.9 g
H. 0.154 mEq
I. 9.99 g

Solutions:

A. 3.50 g of potassium chloride contain

$$3.50 \times \frac{39.1}{74.6} = 1.84 \text{ g of potassium}$$

The formula weight of potassium carbonate is 138.2. 138.2 g of potassium carbonate contain 78.2 g of potassium

$$\frac{78.2}{138.2} = \frac{1.84}{j}$$

$$j = 3.25 \text{ g}$$

B. 5 mL $\times$ 0.1 g/mL = 0.5 g $MgCl_2$

$$MgCl_2 = Mg^{2+} + 2Cl^-$$

Thus 95.3 mg (1 mmol) of $MgCl_2$ yield 2 mmol of Cl^-.

$$\frac{95.3 \text{ mg}}{2 \text{ mmol}} = \frac{500 \text{ mg}}{j}$$

$$j = 10.5 \text{ mmol}$$

C. 1000 g $\times$ 0.0025 = 2.5 g F^-

atomic wt F = 19.0; molecular wt NaF = 42.0

$$\frac{19.0}{42.0} = \frac{2.5 \text{ g}}{j}$$

$$j = 5.53 \text{ g}$$

D. 1 mmol $MgSO_4$ = 120.4 mg = 1 mmol Mg^{2+}

5.0 mmol $\times$ 120.4 mg/mmol = 602 mg = 0.602 g

$$\frac{0.602 \text{ g}}{0.060 \text{ g/mL}} = 10 \text{ mL}$$

E. $15 \text{ mL} \times 0.035 \text{ g/mL} = 0.525 \text{ g}$

   $1 \text{ mmol Cl}^- = 1 \text{ mEq Cl}^- = 1 \text{ mmol KCl} = 74.6 \text{ mg}$

   $$525 \text{ mg} \times \frac{1 \text{ mEq}}{74.6 \text{ mg}} = 7.04 \text{ mEq}$$

F. $MgCl_2 = Mg^{2+} + 2 \text{ Cl}^-$

   $95.3 \text{ mg } (1 \text{ mmol}) \text{ of } MgCl_2 \text{ yield } 2 \text{ mEq of } Mg^{2+}$

   $$20 \text{ mEq} \times \frac{95.3 \text{ mg}}{2 \text{ mEq}} = 953 \text{ mg}$$

   $$\frac{5 \text{ g}}{100 \text{ mL}} = \frac{0.953 \text{ g}}{j}$$

   $j = 19.1 \text{ mL}$

G. $1 \text{ mEq/mL} \times 240 \text{ mL} = 240 \text{ mEq K}^+$

   $K_2SO_4 = 2K^+ + SO_4{}^{2-}$

   $1 \text{ mmol } (174.3 \text{ mg}) \text{ of } K_2SO_4{}^{2-} \text{ yields } 2 \text{ mEq of } K^+$

   $$240 \text{ mEq} \times \frac{174.3 \text{ mg}}{2 \text{ mEq}} = 20,900 \text{ mg} = 20.9 \text{ g}$$

H. Each milliliter contains $1 \text{ mL} \times 0.00900 \text{ g/mL} = 0.00900 \text{ g}$

   $1 \text{ mmol Cl}^- = 1 \text{ mEq Cl}^- = 1 \text{ mmol NaCl} = 58.5 \text{ mg}$

   $$9.00 \text{ mg} \times \frac{1 \text{ mEq}}{58.5 \text{ mg}} = 0.154 \text{ mEq}$$

I. $7.5 \text{ mEq/5 mL} \times 120 \text{ mL} = 180 \text{ mEq}$

   $1 \text{ mmol Ca}^{2+} = 2 \text{ mEq Ca}^{2+} = 1 \text{ mmol CaCl}_2 = 111 \text{ mg}$

   $$180 \text{ mEq} \times \frac{111 \text{ mg}}{2 \text{ mEq}} = 9990 \text{ mg} = 9.99 \text{ g}$$

CHAPTER TEN

OSMOLS AND OSMOLARITY

To prevent irritation and cell destruction when placing a drug solution in contact with a body fluid, the properties of the solution should be matched in certain ways to that of the fluid. To minimize cell damage, the solution should be *isotonic* with the body fluid. Solutions that are injected intravenously (into a vein) should be isotonic with blood. Solutions that are placed in the eye should be isotonic with tears.

An important factor in achieving isotonicity is proper osmotic pressure. Osmotic pressure differences provide the driving force for *osmosis*, the movement of water from regions of low to high solute concentration. Body fluids owe their osmotic pressure to the salts, proteins, and other solutes that are normal components. If a solution that is injected intravenously has too low an osmotic pressure, water will flow into red blood cells, causing them to swell. If the osmotic pressure is too high, the cells will lose water and become shrunken. Movement of fluid into or out of cells is minimized when the drug solution that is introduced has the same osmotic pressure as that of the fluid. Such solutions are said to be *isoosmotic* with the particular fluid.

Osmotic pressure is a major determinant of tonicity but it is not the only one. Solutions containing certain drugs can damage red blood cells despite the fact that they have the correct osmotic pressure. Nevertheless, monitoring osmotic pressure is a necessary step in assuring isotonicity.

Although the osmotic pressure of a solution can be determined (using an instrument called an *osmometer*), calculated theoretical values are helpful in estimating whether a solution's osmotic pressure is likely to be in the correct range of values. In this chapter, we explore the units used to designate osmotic pressure. You will learn to calculate the theoretical contribution made by solutes to osmotic pressure of solutions.

Learning objectives: after completing this chapter the student should be able to

1. State the number of milliosmols contributed by a given quantity of an electrolyte or nonelectrolyte.
2. Calculate theoretical osmolarity or osmolality from a knowledge of the quantities of solute(s) used to prepare a solution.
3. Convert percentage strength of a solute to osmolar units.

---

1. Osmotic pressure is one of the colligative properties. Like freezing point depression and boiling point elevation by dissolved solids, osmotic pressure depends only on the number of particles (molecules or ions) dissolved in unit volume of solvent. When an ideally behaving nonelectrolyte is dissolved in water, each molecule produces one particle in solution. For real substances, the same holds true provided that there is no dimerization or polymerization of molecules in solution.

    The number of particles is expressed in terms of osmols. One osmol (Osm) is defined as the weight, in grams, of a solute osmotically equivalent to one gram-molecular weight (1 mol) of an ideally behaving nonelectrolyte. A milliosmol (mOsm) is 1/1000 of an osmol.

    One mole (gram-molecular weight) of an ideal nonelectrolyte is equivalent to 1 osmol and 1 milliequivalent equals 1 milliosmol. Consequently, 1 mOsm of a nonelectrolyte is equivalent to the molecular weight expressed in milligrams. In terms of equations, for ideal nonelectrolytes,

    1 Osm = 1 mol

    1 mOsm = 0.001 Osm = 1 mmol

    Consider sucrose (sugar), whose molecular weight is 342. 342 g represent 1 mol of sucrose; theoretically, 342 g also represent 1 Osm of sucrose. Calculate the theoretical number of osmols and milliosmols equivalent to 1 g of sucrose.

0.00292 Osm; 2.92 mOsm

Solution:

$$1 \text{ Osm} = 342 \text{ g}$$

$$1 \text{ g} \times \frac{1 \text{ Osm}}{342} = 0.00292 \text{ Osm}$$

$$0.00292 \text{ Osm} \times \frac{1000 \text{ mOsm}}{1 \text{ Osm}} = 2.92 \text{ mOsm}$$

---

2. How many grams of dextrose, molecular weight 180, would be needed to provide 120 mOsm?

— — — — — — — — — — — — — — — — — — — —

21.6 g

Solution:

$$1 \text{ mOsm} = 180 \text{ mg (molecular weight expressed in mg)}$$

$$120 \text{ mOsm} \times \frac{180 \text{ mg}}{1 \text{ mOsm}} = 21,600 \text{ mg} = 21.6 \text{ g}$$

---

3. We can calculate the theoretical number of osmols or milliosmols of electrolytes by taking the number of ions formed into consideration. In this and all the other examples to follow, water is the only solvent considered because of the application to biological fluids. For purposes of calculation the number of osmols is taken to be the sum of the number of moles produced by complete ionization. We must recognize that the number of osmols resulting from putting an electrolyte into solution will be less than the theoretical value if dissociation is not complete. However, the assumption of complete dissociation is a good one for many salts of clinical importance and the theoretical value is close to the measured value. As an example, sodium chloride dissociates into two ions:

$$NaCl = Na^+ + Cl^-$$

From the equation above, we can see that 1 mol of NaCl dissociates to yield 2 mol of ions. Each mole of ions represents particles that contribute to the osmotic pressure. Each mole of the ions produced adds another osmol. In other words,

1 mol NaCl = 2 Osm (1 Osm Na^+ + 1 Osm Cl^-)

Since the formula weight of NaCl is 58.5,

58.5 g of NaCl = 2 Osm and 58.5 mg = 2 mOsm of NaCl

Calculate the number of theoretical milliosmols corresponding to 0.386 g of NaCl.

_ _ _ _ _ _ _ _ _ _ _ _ _ _ _ _ _ _ _ _

13.2 mOsm

Solution:

1 mol = 58.5 g NaCl = 2 Osm

1 mmol = 58.5 mg NaCl = 2 mOsm

$$386 \text{ mg} \times \frac{2 \text{ mOsm}}{58.5 \text{ mg}} = 13.2 \text{ mOsm}$$

4. How many grams of calcium chloride would produce 100 mOsm?

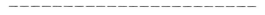

3.7 g

Solution:

$$CaCl_2 = Ca^{2+} + 2\ Cl^-$$

From the equation, each mole of $CaCl_2$ yields 3 Osm. The formula weight of $CaCl_2$ is 111. Therefore,

$$111\ g\ CaCl_2 = 3\ Osm;\ 111\ mg\ CaCl_2 = 3\ mOsm$$

$$100\ mOsm\ \times \frac{111\ mg}{3\ mOsm} = 3700\ mg = 3.7\ g$$

---

5.   Recall that water of hydration present within a crystal becomes part of the solvent when the solid is dissolved in water. It affects the molecular weight of the solid, but not the number of osmols in solution. (The water of hydration contributes no particles.) How many grams of $CaCl_2 \cdot 2H_2O$ would produce 100 mOsm?

- -

4.9 g. Note that the amount required is larger than for the anhydrous salt (see frame 4).

Solution:

$$CaCl_2 \cdot 2H_2O = Ca^{2+} + 2Cl^- + 2H_2O$$

$$147\ mg\ CaCl_2 \cdot 2H_2O = 3\ mOsm\ \text{(the water adds no particles)}$$

$$100\ mOsm\ \times \frac{147\ mg}{3\ mOsm} = 4900\ mg = 4.9\ g$$

---

6.   How many milliosmols of calcium ion are there in 8.75 g of anhydrous calcium chloride?

78.5 mOsm

Solution:

$$CaCl_2 = Ca^{2+} + 2Cl^-$$

The equation shows that each mole of $CaCl_2$ produces 1 mol of Ca^{2+}. Consequently, 111 mg of $CaCl_2$ yield 1 mOsm of Ca^{2+}.

$$8750 \text{ mg} \times \frac{1 \text{ mOsm } Ca^{2+}}{111 \text{ mg}} = 78.5 \text{ mOsm } Ca^{2+}$$

---

7. It is the concentration of osmols in solution rather than the absolute number, that determines osmotic pressure. So while it is important to be able to calculate the number of osmols (or milliosmols) contributed by a solute, it is also necessary to know how to determine osmol concentration. Two common expressions for osmol concentration are used; they are osmolarity and osmolality.

    Osmolarity is analogous to molarity. In fact, for nonelectrolytes, they are numerically the same. A 1-osmolar solution contains 1 Osm per liter of solution. If 2 Osm are present in a liter, we have a 2 osmolar solution. If 150 mOsm are dissolved in enough water to make a liter, the solution is 150 milliosmolar. More commonly, this concentration would simply be expressed as 150 mOsm/L. Osmolarity is a weight/volume type of situation in which the amount of solute and volume of total solution are specified.

    The second unit is *osmolality*. A 1-osmolal solution contains 1 osmol per kilogram of water. For practical purposes, the density of water can be taken as 1 g/ml, so that 1 kg = 1 L. If 300 mOsm are dissolved in a liter of water, the solution is 300 milliosmolal.

    For each of the following examples, calculate the concentration (either osmolarity or osmolality as appropriate) and tell which it is.

A. 22 mOsm dissolved in 100 mL of water.
B. 15 mOsm dissolved in enough water to make a total volume of 100 mL.
C. A solution containing 0.25 mOsm/mL of solution.
D. A solution containing 0.20 mOsm/mL of water.

A. 220 milliosmolal or 0.22 osmolal
B. 150 milliosmolar or 0.15 osmolar

C.   250 milliosmolar or 0.25 osmolar
D.   200 milliosmolal or 0.2 osmolal

---

8.   Why have two sets of units? Osmolarity is useful because solutions are conveniently administered by volume and we want to know what quantity of components are contained within any given volume. This fits right in with a w/v arrangement. On the other hand, osmotic pressure is a function of osmolal concentration and instrumental measurements are better related to osmolal values than the osmolar designation.

For dilute solutions, the difference between osmolar and osmolal concentrations is usually very small. This is because the solute occupies so little space in the solution that the volume of the solvent is almost the same as the solution's total volume. In such cases only, it is possible to make the approximation that osmolality and osmolarity are numerically equal. As an example, the osmolality and osmolarity of a 0.9% solution of sodium chloride differ by less than 1%. However, equating osmolality and osmolarity is not valid when dealing with concentrated systems.

For which of the following solutions are osmolality and osmolarity most likely to have a similar value?

A.   10% fructose solution
B.   0.1% dextrose solution

B is correct. The solute concentration is small enough so that the contribution of solute to total volume is negligible.

---

9.   Let's try an example to see how osmolarity is calculated using dextrose as a solute. If we make 400 mL of a solution containing 30.0 g of hydrous dextrose (MW = 198), its concentration can be calculated as follows:

For dextrose, 1 mol = 1 Osm = 198 g.

$$30.0 \text{ g} \times \frac{1 \text{ mol}}{198 \text{ g}} = 0.152 \text{ mol} = 0.152 \text{ Osm} = 152 \text{ mOsm}$$

$$\frac{152 \text{ mOsm}}{400 \text{ mL}} = \frac{j}{1000 \text{ mL}}$$

$$j = 380 \text{ mOsm/L}$$

Calculate the concentration, in mOsm/L, of a 5% w/v solution prepared by dissolving hydrous dextrose in water.

---

253 mOsm/L

Solution:

5% = 5 g/100 mL = 50 g/L

$$50 \text{ g/L} \times \frac{1 \text{ Osm}}{198 \text{ g}} = 0.253 \text{ Osm/L} = 253 \text{ mOsm/L}$$

The concentration is 253 mOsm/L. Alternately, recognizing that a 1 Osm solution contains 198 g/L,

198 g/L:1 Osm/L = 50 g/L:j

j = 0.253 Osm/L or 253 mOsm/L

---

10. Calculate the concentration, in mOsm/L, of a 0.9% solution of sodium chloride in water.

---

308 mOsm/L

Solution:

$NaCl = Na^+ + Cl^-$

1 mmol NaCl = 58.5 mg NaCl = 2 mOsm

0.9% = 0.9 g/100 mL = 9 g/L = 9000 mg/L

$$9000 \text{ mg/L} \times \frac{2 \text{ mOsm}}{58.5 \text{ mg}} = 308 \text{ mOsm/L}$$

---

11. Calculate the number of grams of potassium chloride needed to make 200 mL of a solution to theoretically contain 250 mOsm/L.

1.87 g

Solution:

$$KCl = K^+ + Cl^-$$

1 mmol KCl (74.6 mg) is equivalent to 2 mOsm.

250 mOsm/L $\times$ 0.2 L = 50 mOsm needed.

$$50 \text{ mOsm} \times \frac{74.6 \text{ mg}}{2 \text{ mOsm}} = 1870 \text{ mg} = 1.87 \text{ g}$$

12. How many theoretical milliosmols of sodium ion are there in each milliliter of a 1% solution of sodium sulfate? How many theoretical milliosmols total?

0.141 mOsm Na$^+$/mL; a total of 0.211 mOsm/mL

Solution:

$$Na_2SO_4 \text{ (142 g/mol)} = 2Na^+ + SO4^{2-}$$

1 mmol (142 mg) = 2 mOsm Na$^+$ + 1 mOsm SO4^{2-}

A 1% solution contains 1 g/100 mL = 0.01 g/mL = 10 mg/mL.

For Na$^+$:

$$10 \text{ mg salt/mL} \times \frac{2 \text{ mOsm Na}^+}{142 \text{ mg}} = 0.141 \text{ mOsm Na}^+/\text{mL}$$

Total:

$$10 \text{ mg salt/mL} \times \frac{3 \text{ mOsm}}{142 \text{ mg}} = 0.211 \text{ mOsm/mL}$$

---

13. In some instances, the quantity of solute contributing to the osmolarity of a solution is expressed in millimoles or milliequivalents instead of a mass unit. For nonelectrolytes, each millimole theoretically contributes 1 milliosmol to a solution. For electrolytes, the number of milliosmols per millimole can easily be determined by inspection of the dissociation equation.

    As an example, let us calculate the number of theoretical milliosmols per 100 mL of a solution containing 14 mmol of dextrose and 2.0 mmol of potassium chloride per 100 mL.

Dextrose:

    14 mmol = 14 mOsm

KCl:

    $KCl = K^+ + Cl^-$;

    2 mOsm = 1 mmol ; 2 mmol = 4 mOsm

Total: 14 mOsm + 4 mOsm = 18 mOsm/100 mL

    Calculate the number of theoretical mOsm/mL in a solution containing 130 mmol/L sodium chloride and 30 mmol/L magnesium chloride.

- -

0.35 mOsm/mL

Solution:

    $NaCl = Na^+ + Cl^-$; 1 mmol = 2 mOsm

    $MgCl_2 = Mg^{2+} + 2Cl^-$; 1 mmol = 3 mOsm

$$NaCl: 130 \text{ mmol/L} \times \frac{2 \text{ mOsm}}{1 \text{ mmol}} = 260 \text{ mOsm/L}$$

$$MgCl_2: 30 \text{ mmol/L} \times \frac{3 \text{ mOsm}}{1 \text{ mmol}} = 90 \text{ mOsm/L}$$

$$260 + 90 = 350 \text{ mOsm/L} = 0.35 \text{ mOsm/mL}$$

---

14. How many theoretical milliosmols/L are there in 1 L of a NaCl solution containing 1 mEq of sodium ion in each 20 mL?

_____

100 mOsm

Solution:

$$NaCl = Na^+ + Cl^-$$

From the equation, each millimole of NaCl contributes 1 mEq of sodium ion and a total of 2 mOsm to the solution. This solution contains 2 mOsm for each mEq of Na^+. Consequently, 20 mL contain 2 mOsm, 100 mL contain 10 mOsm and a liter contains 100 mOsm.

---

15. In frame 10 we saw that normal saline solution, 0.9 g NaCl per 100 mL, had an osmolarity of 308 mOsm/L. If a solution is injected intravenously, it should have close to the same osmolarity (within about a 10% tolerance) to avoid cell destruction and tissue damage. If a small volume is injected slowly, minimal disruption occurs because it is diluted by plasma. However, injection of large volumes with incorrect osmolarity can cause problems. We can use calculations of theoretical osmolarity to get an idea of whether an osmotic pressure imbalance is likely. As an example, let us calculate the theoretical osmolarity of Ringer's solution, a salt solution that may be injected for fluid replacement or as a means of drug administration. Ringer's solution contains 0.86% sodium chloride, 0.03% potassium chloride and 0.033% calcium chloride. The respective formula weights are 58.5, 74.6 and 111.

Verify by writing the dissociation equations that each millimole is equivalent to 2 mOsm in the case of NaCl and KCl and that for $CaCl_2$, each millimole is equivalent to 3 mOsm.

NaCl: 0.86 g/100 mL = 860 mg/100 mL = 8,600 mg/L

$$8600 \text{ mg/L} \times \frac{1 \text{ mmoL}}{58.5 \text{ mg}} \times \frac{2 \text{ mOsm}}{1 \text{ mmol}} = 294 \text{ mOsm/L}$$

$$\text{KCl: } 300 \text{ mg/L} \times \frac{1 \text{ mmoL}}{74.6 \text{ mg}} \times \frac{2 \text{ mOsm}}{1 \text{ mmol}} = 8.04 \text{ mOsm/L}$$

$$CaCl_2\text{: } 330 \text{ mg/L} \times \frac{1 \text{ mmoL}}{111 \text{ mg}} \times \frac{3 \text{ mOsm}}{1 \text{ mmol}} = 8.92 \text{ mOsm/L}$$

The total is 311 mOsm/L, which is quite close to the value of 308 mOsm/L for normal saline solution. Therefore, Ringer's solution is osmotically equivalent to normal saline solution.

Calculate the theoretical osmolarity of a solution containing 2.5% dextrose (MW = 198) and 0.45% sodium chloride and compare it to normal saline solution.

----

280 mOsm/L. This is osmotically equivalent to normal saline solution.

Solution:

$$\text{Dextrose: } 25,000 \text{ mg/L} \times \frac{1 \text{ mOsm}}{198 \text{ mg}} = 126 \text{ mOsm/L}$$

$$\text{NaCl: } 4500 \text{ mg/L} \times \frac{2 \text{ mOsm}}{58.5 \text{ mg}} = 154 \text{ mOsm/L}$$

The total is 280 mOsm/L which is within 10% of normal saline solution and so is osmotically equivalent.

16. Do all of these problems before verifying your answers.

A. Calculate the number of theoretical milliosmols in 350 mL of normal saline solution.

B. If the osmotic pressure of a potassium chloride solution is expressed as 220 mOsm/L , what is its percentage strength?

C. Calculate the number of theoretical mOsm/L in a solution containing 5% dextrose (MW = 198) and 0.2% sodium chloride.

D. How many grams of $CaCl_2 \cdot 2H_2O$ should be dissolved in water to make 150 mL of a solution that contains 298 mOsm/L?

- -

A. 108 mOsm
B. 0.821%
C. 321 mOsm/L
D. 2.19 g

Solutions:

A. $350 \text{ mL} \times \dfrac{900 \text{ mg}}{100 \text{ mL}} \times \dfrac{2 \text{ mOsm}}{58.5 \text{ mg}} = 108 \text{ mOsm}$

B. $220 \text{ mOsm} \times \dfrac{74.6 \text{ mg}}{2 \text{mOsm}} = 8210 \text{ mg/L}$

    $= 0.821 \text{ g/100 mL or } 0.821\%$

C. Dextrose: $50{,}000 \text{ mg/L} \times \dfrac{1 \text{ mOsm}}{198 \text{ mg}} = 253 \text{ mOsm/L}$

$$\text{NaCl: } 2000 \text{ mg/L} \times \frac{2 \text{ mOsm}}{58.5 \text{ mg}} = 68 \text{ mOsm/L}$$

Total = 321 mOsm/L

D. $CaCl_2 \cdot 2H_2O = Ca^{2+} + 2Cl^- + 2H_2O$

147 mg $CaCl_2 \cdot 2H_2O$ = 3 mOsm

$$0.150 \text{ L} \times 298 \text{ mOsm/L} \times \frac{0.147 \text{ g}}{3 \text{ mOsm}} = 2.19 \text{ g}$$

CHAPTER ELEVEN

ISOOSMOTIC SOLUTIONS

In Chapter 10 we saw that osmotic pressure is an important characteristic of liquids that come in contact with blood, tears, or other body fluids. The importance of osmotic pressure as a means of avoiding irritation and cell damage was emphasized. In this chapter we explore ways of adjusting osmotic pressure by the addition of sodium chloride or other compounds to solutions whose osmotic pressure is too low.

Learning objectives: after completing this chapter the student should be able to

1. Determine the sodium chloride equivalent of a substance from the volume of isotonic solution that can be made from 1 g of that substance.
2. Apply the sodium chloride equivalent method to determine the amount of NaCl needed to make a solution isoosmotic with body fluids.
3. Apply the sodium chloride equivalent method to determine the amount of a substance other than sodium chloride needed to make a solution isoosmotic with body fluids.

---

1. The osmotic pressure of a solution depends on the number of ions and molecules that are dissolved. Other properties that depend on the number of microparticles in solution are freezing point depression and boiling point elevation. These are called *colligative properties*. As they are all related to each other, freezing point

---

depression has often been used as a means of estimating the effect of solutes on osmotic pressure. Blood serum and the fluid bathing the eye freeze at –0.52°C. A 0.9% solution of sodium chloride in water, often referred to as *normal saline solution*, also freezes at –0.52°C and is isoosmotic with these fluids. It follows that other water solutions that freeze at –0.52°C will also be isoosmotic.

A. How many milligrams of NaCl are found in each milliliter of normal saline solution?
B. How many grams of NaCl are there in 120 mL of normal saline solution?

A. 9 mg
B. 1.08 g

Solutions:

$$1 \text{ mL} \times \frac{0.9 \text{ g}}{100 \text{ mL}} = 0.009 \text{ g} = 9 \text{ mg}$$

$$120 \text{ mL} \times \frac{0.9 \text{ g}}{100 \text{ mL}} = 1.08 \text{ g}$$

2. Most often, simple solutions of drugs at therapeutic concentrations in water have an osmotic pressure that is too small. It is necessary to add another material (usually sodium chloride is chosen) to make the solution isoosmotic with body fluids. Why is sodium chloride a reasonable choice for adjusting osmotic pressure? Both sodium and chloride are predominant ions in biological fluids, so this salt does not cause irritation or otherwise disturb normal processes. There are several ways of calculating the amount of sodium chloride that should be used. We will discuss only one of them: the method of sodium chloride equivalents.

For a particular drug, there is a single concentration at which the drug solution will be isoosmotic with blood serum and tears. If we start with 1 g of drug, it will be possible to prepare a certain volume of isoosmotic solution, depending on the isoosmotic concentration. The USP has a table (under the heading

"Ophthalmic Solutions") listing the volume of isoosmotic solution that can be made from 1 g of several drugs.

From the table, 14.3 mL of isoosmotic solution in water can be prepared from 1 g of atropine sulfate. Recalling that 0.9% aqueous sodium chloride solution is isoosmotic, the amount of sodium chloride in 14.3 mL would be

$$14.3 \text{ mL} \times 0.009 \text{ g/mL} = 0.13 \text{ g NaCl}$$

Thus 14.3 mL of an isoosmotic solution of atropine sulfate contain 1 g of atropine sulfate while 14.3 mL of an isoosmotic solution of sodium chloride contain 0.13 g of NaCl. Therefore, 0.13 g of NaCl generates the same osmotic pressure as 1 g of atropine sulfate. In terms of osmotic pressure, each gram of atropine sulfate can be replaced by 0.13 g of NaCl. 0.13 is called the *sodium chloride equivalent* of atropine sulfate.

7.7 mL of a solution containing 1 g of streptomycin sulfate is isoosmotic with tears. Calculate the sodium chloride equivalent of streptomycin sulfate.

————————————————————————

0.069 g

Solution:

For isotonic sodium chloride solution,

$$7.7 \text{ mL} \times \frac{0.9 \text{ g}}{100 \text{ mL}} = 0.069 \text{ g NaCl}$$

Therefore, 0.069 g of NaCl is osmotically equivalent to 1 g of streptomycin sulfate; 0.069 is the sodium chloride equivalent of this drug.

3. Other sodium chloride equivalents can be calculated from the table in the USP. Rather complete tables listing sodium chloride equivalents can also be found in several reference sources, such as Remington's Pharmaceutical Sciences.

    Let us try a problem that shows how sodium chloride equivalents can be put to work. It is necessary to prepare 300 mL of a 1.0% solution of atropine sulfate. How many grams of sodium chloride should be dissolved in the solution to make it isoosmotic with tears?

If no atropine sulfate were present, the amount of sodium chloride needed for isotonicity would be

$$300 \text{ mL} \times 0.009 \text{ g/mL} = 2.70 \text{ g}$$

However, the solution does contain

$$300 \text{ mL} \times 0.01 \text{ g/mL} = 3.0 \text{ g atropine sulfate}$$

This amount of atropine sulfate exerts a certain osmotic pressure. Using the sodium chloride equivalent (0.13), we can determine the amount of sodium chloride that has the same osmotic pressure as 3.0 g of atropine sulfate:

$$3.0 \text{ g} \times 0.13 = 0.39 \text{ g NaCl}$$

The atropine sulfate in the solution exerts an osmotic pressure equal to that of 0.39 g of NaCl. Therefore, to find the amount of sodium chloride to add, it is necessary to subtract 0.39 g from the amount of NaCl that would have been needed had the salt been the only solute in the system.

$$2.70 \text{ g} - 0.39 \text{ g} = 2.31 \text{ g}$$

To prepare the solution, dissolve 3 g of atropine sulfate and 2.31 g of a sodium chloride in sufficient water to make a total volume of 300 mL.

To recapitulate, follow these three steps:

(1) Calculate the number of grams of NaCl needed to make the desired volume isoosmotic.

(2) Using values of the respective sodium chloride equivalents, calculate the amount of NaCl osmotically equivalent to each of the other formula components and total these.

(3) Subtract the result in (2) from (1) to yield the amount of NaCl that must be used.

How many grams of sodium chloride should be used to make 90 mL of a 0.5% pilocarpine hydrochloride solution isoosmotic? The sodium chloride equivalent for pilocarpine hydrochloride is 0.24.

0.702 g

Solution:

90 mL × 0.5 g/100 mL = 0.45 g pilocarpine hydrochloride

Step 1:   90 mL × 0.009 g/mL = 0.81 g NaCl

Step 2:   0.45 g × 0.24 = 0.108 g NaCl

Step 3:   0.81 g − 0.108 g = 0.702 g NaCl

---

4.   Here is another problem:

℞

Phenylephrine HCl	0.25%
Zinc sulfate	0.5%
Sodium chloride qs	
Purified water, qs ad	60.0 mL

How many grams of sodium chloride should be used to make this solution isoosmotic? (The sodium chloride equivalent of phenylephrine hydrochloride is 0.32; that of zinc sulfate is 0.15.)

0.093 g

Solution:

If NaCl were the only solute, the amount needed would be

60.0 mL × 0.009 g/mL = 0.54 g

For phenylephrine HCl:

60 mL × 0.0025 g/mL = 0.15 g

0.15 g × 0.32 = 0.048 g NaCl

For zinc sulfate:

$$60 \text{ mL} \times 0.005 \text{ g/mL} = 0.3 \text{ g}$$

$$0.3 \text{ g} \times 0.15 = 0.045 \text{ g NaCl}$$

The total amount of sodium chloride equivalent to the osmotic pressure exerted by both drugs is

$$0.048 \text{ g} + 0.045 \text{ g} = 0.093 \text{ g NaCl}$$

The amount of sodium chloride needed is

$$0.54 \text{ g} - 0.093 \text{ g} = 0.447 \text{ g}$$

To make the solution, dissolve 0.15 g of phenylephrine hydrochloride, 0.3 g of zinc sulfate, and 0.447 g of sodium chloride in sufficient water to make 60 mL.

---

5. How much sodium chloride should be included in 1 L of solution containing 1% gentamycin sulfate and 1:1000 benzalkonium chloride? Sodium chloride equivalents: gentamycin sulfate, 0.05; benzalkonium chloride, 0.16.

- -

8.34 g

Solution:

$$1000 \text{ mL} \times 0.009 \text{ g/mL} = 9 \text{ g NaCl}$$

Gentamycin sulfate: $1000 \text{ mL} \times 1 \text{ g/100 mL} \times 0.05 = 0.5 \text{ g}$

Benzalkonium chloride: $1000 \text{ mL} \times 1 \text{ g/1000 mL} \times 0.16 = 0.16 \text{ g}$

$$9 \text{ g} - (0.5 + 0.16) \text{ g} = 8.34 \text{ g NaCl needed}$$

---

6. Sometimes, an agent other than sodium chloride may be used to adjust osmotic pressure. Silver salts would precipitate in the presence of chloride ion, so another salt such as sodium nitrate

might be used. Boric acid is sometimes used in place of sodium chloride in solutions used in the eye. If a substance other than sodium chloride is to be employed to raise osmotic pressure, the calculation procedure requires one extra step.

To begin, follow the same procedure as though sodium chloride were to be used. After calculating the amount of sodium chloride needed, divide that amount by the sodium chloride equivalent of the substance that will be used to raise the osmotic pressure of the solution. This produces the required result.

As an example, let us calculate the amount of sodium nitrate needed to make 200 mL of a 0.6% solution of silver nitrate isoosmotic. The sodium chloride equivalent of silver nitrate is 0.33. That of sodium nitrate is 0.68. If only sodium chloride were present, the amount needed would be

$$200 \text{ mL} \times 0.009 \text{ g/mL} = 1.8 \text{ g NaCl}$$

The amount of silver nitrate needed is

$$200 \text{ mL} \times 0.6 \text{ g/100 mL} = 1.2 \text{ g}$$

This is osmotically equivalent to

$$1.2 \times 0.33 = 0.396 \text{ g NaCl}$$

The amount of sodium chloride that would have to be added is

$$1.8 \text{ g} - 0.396 \text{ g} = 1.404 \text{ g NaCl}$$

To find the amount of sodium nitrate that should be used to adjust osmotic pressure, we divide by the sodium chloride equivalent of that substance.

$$\frac{1.404}{0.68} = 2.06 \text{ g NaNO}_3$$

Calculate the amount of boric acid that should be included in 300 mL of a 0.4% procaine hydrochloride solution to render the solution isoosmotic. Sodium chloride equivalents: procaine hydrochloride, 0.21; boric acid, 0.50.

4.9 g

Solution:

> 300 mL × 0.009 g/mL = 2.7 g NaCl
>
> 300 mL × 0.4 g/100 mL = 1.2 g procaine hydrochloride
>
> 1.2 × 0.21 = 0.252 g NaCl
>
> 2.7 g − 0.252 g = 2.45 g NaCl needed
>
> $\dfrac{2.45\ g}{0.5}$ = 4.9 g boric acid

---

7. Do all of the following problems before verifying your answers.

A.   ℞

   Cocaine hydrochloride   1.2 g
   Sodium chloride qs
   Purified water qs ad   30 mL

   How much sodium chloride should be used to make this eye solution isoosmotic (isotonic)? The sodium chloride equivalent of cocaine hydrochloride is 0.16.

B.   A pharmacist has to prepare 500 mL of a 1% solution of procaine hydrochloride for use in the eye. How many grams of sodium chloride should be used to make the solution isoosmotic with tears? The sodium chloride equivalent of procaine hydrochloride is 0.21.

C.   A solution for use as an eyedrop is to contain 0.4 g of ephedrine sulfate and 1 g of tetracycline hydrochloride per 100 mL. How many grams of sodium chloride must each 100 mL of the solution contain if it is to be isoosmotic with tears? Sodium chloride equivalent of ephedrine sulfate is 0.23; that of tetracycline hydrochloride is 0.14.

D. A pharmacist has to prepare 30 mL of 1% tetracaine hydrochloride solution. How much boric acid should be used to make this solution isoosmotic? The sodium chloride equivalent of tetracaine hydrochloride is 0.18; the sodium chloride equivalent of boric acid is 0.50.

E. The formula for an ophthalmic solution contains:

Ingredient X	1.5 %
Zinc sulfate	0.2 %
Sodium chloride	
Water, sufficient to make	100%

Calculate the amount of sodium chloride required to render 1.50 L of the solution isotonic. Sodium chloride equivalents: ingredient X: 0.22; zinc sulfate: 0.16.

F. ℞

Atropine sulfate	1.2 %
Boric acid qs	
Purified water qs ad	15 mL

M. ft. opth. sol.

The sodium chloride equivalents are atropine sulf.: 0.13; boric acid: 0.50. Calculate the amount of boric acid needed to make this solution isotonic.

––––––––––––––––––––––––

A. 0.078 g NaCl
B. 3.45 g NaCl
C. 0.668 g NaCl
D. 0.432 g boric acid
E. 8.07 g NaCl
F. 0.224 g boric acid

Solutions:

A. 30 mL × 0.009 g/mL = 0.27 g NaCl

   1.2 g × 0.16 = 0.192 g

   0.27 − 0.192 g = 0.078 g NaCl needed

B. 500 mL × 0.009 g/mL = 4.5 g NaCl

   5 g procaine HCl × 0.21 = 1.05 g NaCl

   4.5 g NaCl − 1.05 g NaCl = 3.45 g NaCl needed

C. 100 mL requires 0.9 g NaCl for isotonicity

   e.s.: 0.4 g × 0.23 = 0.092 g NaCl

   t.h.: 1 g × 0.14 = 0.14 g NaCl

   0.9 g − (0.092 + 0.14) g = 0.668 g NaCl needed

D. 30 mL × 0.009 g/mL = 0.27 g NaCl

   30 mL × 1 g/100 mL = 0.3 g t.h.

   0.3 g × 0.18 = 0.054 g NaCl

   0.27 g − 0.054 g = 0.216 g NaCl needed

   $\dfrac{0.216\ g}{0.50}$ = 0.432 g boric acid

E. NaCl alone: 1500 mL × 0.009 g/mL = 13.5 g

   Ingredient X: 1500 mL × 1.5 g/100 mL = 22.5 g

   22.5 g × 0.22 = 4.95 g NaCl

Zinc sulfate: 1500×0.2 g/100 mL = 3 g

3 g $\times$ 0.16 = 0.48 g NaCl

13.5 g NaCl – (4.95 g + 0.48 g) = 8.07 g NaCl

F. NaCl alone: 15 mL $\times$ 0.009 g/mL = 0.135 g

Atropine sulfate: 15 mL $\times$ 1.2 g/100 mL = 0.18 g

0.18 g $\times$ 0.13 = 0.023 g NaCl

0.135 g – 0.023 = 0.112 g NaCl

$\dfrac{0.112\ g}{0.50}$ = 0.224 g boric acid

CHAPTER TWELVE

PARENTERAL NUTRITION

In recent years, the practice of feeding by slow intravenous administration has become established. One application of this technique is the treatment of malnourished persons or those unable to eat or digest food. Even otherwise normal patients may require intravenous feeding following traumatic injury, such as an auto accident, because the body temporarily uses stored energy faster than three square meals can replace it.

The term *parenteral* identifies administration by a route other than oral. Parenteral nutrition may utilize one of the large, central veins, a smaller peripheral vein, or both. The patient may be totally reliant on intravenous administration for nutrition. The term *TPN*, which stands for *total parenteral nutrition*, is frequently used to describe a mixture that is expected to supply all needed fluid, electrolytes, calories, essential fatty acids, and vitamins— in short, everything needed to sustain life.

Many books and articles on this subject have been published. The following were used as references for the information in this chapter:
1. Total Parenteral Nutrition in the Hospital and at Home, K. N. Jeejeebhoy (Ed.), CRC Press, Boca Raton, 1983.
2. J. P. Grant, Handbook of Total Parenteral Nutrition, 2nd edition, W. B. Saunders, Philadelphia, 1992.
3. Total Parenteral Nutrition, edited by J. E. Fischer (Ed.), Little, Brown, Boston, 1991.

Identification of patients who are candidates for parenteral nutrition, selection of nutrients and other topics of obvious importance are not covered in this chapter. We concentrate on many of the calculations that have to be performed in connection with parenteral nutrition.

Learning objectives: after completing this chapter the student should be able to

1. Calculate the volume of a stock solution that will supply a needed quantity of electrolyte, carbohydrate, fat or other nutrient.
2. Determine the caloric content of a specified volume of a carbohydrate or fat preparation.
3. Determine the amount of nitrogen present in a given volume of an amino acid solution.
4. Calculate the ratio between nonprotein calories and nitrogen in a parenteral mixture.

---

1. In preparing solutions for nutrition, the pharmacist makes extensive use of commercial products. These are typically solutions or dispersions in which each unit of volume contains known amounts of essential electrolytes or nutrient components. Products containing hydrolyzed protein or amino acids are given to provide the building blocks for protein manufacture.

    As an example, a TPN solution is to contain 4% amino acids. The source is a commercial product that contains 10 g of amino acids per 100 mL. Let's say that we wish to prepare 1 L of the TPN solution. We have to calculate the amount of source product to use. A simple approach is to begin with a mass balance equation. In the equation, aa stands for amino acids.

    let j = volume of amino acid source to be used

    amount of aa in source = amount of aa in TPN

    $j \times 10$ g/100 mL = 1000 mL $\times$ 4 g/100 mL

    $j = 400$ mL

    How many milliliters of the same amino acid source product would be needed to prepare 2.5 L of a TPN solution containing 4.2% amino acids?

1050 mL

Solution:

$j \times 10$ g/100 mL = 2500 mL $\times 4.2$ g/100 mL

$j = 1050$ mL

---

2. A TPN solution is to contain sodium, 60 mEq/L and calcium, 9 mEq/L. A sodium chloride solution with a concentration of 4 mEq/mL is available. How much of this solution is needed to contribute the sodium ion in preparing 2 L of the TPN solution?

_ _

30 mL

Solution:

$j \times 4$ mEq/mL = 2 L $\times 60$ mEq/L

$j = 30$ mL

---

3. Referring to frame 2, how many milliliters of a calcium gluconate solution containing 0.45 mEq/mL of calcium ion should be used to prepare 2 L of the TPN solution?

_ _

40 mL

Solution:

$j \times 0.45$ mEq/mL = 2 L $\times 9$ mEq/L

$j = 40$ mL

4. Calculate the quantity of KCl solution, 2 mEq/mL, needed to supply potassium ion in 1.75 L of a solution to contain 40 mEq of potassium ion/liter.

———————————————————————

35 mL

Solution:

$$j \times 2 \text{ mEq/mL} = 1.75 \text{ L} \times 40 \text{ mEq/L}$$

$$j = 35 \text{ mL}$$

5. One liter of a parenteral nutrition mixture is to contain 8 mEq of calcium ion and 100 mEq of chloride. Other electrolyte solutions that have been used have already supplied 95 mEq of chloride. Our problem is to decide what combination of calcium gluconate, 0.45 mEq/mL, and calcium chloride, 1.36 mEq/mL should be used.

First, let us recall that each electrolyte yields the same number of mEq of cation and anion. Therefore, the calcium chloride solution contains 1.36 mEq/mL of chloride also.

Next, we have to decide which ion, Ca^{2+} or Cl^-, is needed in smallest quantity. If it is the calcium, we can get all of this ion from the calcium chloride stock solution which will also supply some of the chloride, and use another salt to contribute the remaining chloride. If the chloride is needed in smallest quantity, then we add enough calcium chloride stock to supply the chloride and just part of the calcium. The gluconate stock solution is used to contribute the remaining calcium ion. In this case, we need 8 mEq of Ca^{2+} and 5 mEq of Cl^-. Can you determine what quantity of each stock solution to add?

———————————————————————

3.68 mL of CaCl$_2$ stock; 6.67 mL of gluconate stock

Solution:

For chloride, 100 mEq − 95 mEq = 5 mEq remain

$j \times 1.36$ mEq/mL = 5 mEq

$j = 3.68$ mL of calcium chloride stock

This stock solution contributes 5 mEq of chloride ion and 5 mEq of calcium ion. That means that we still need 3 mEq of calcium, which will come from the gluconate stock:

$j \times 0.45$ mEq/mL = 3 mEq

$j = 6.67$ mL of calcium gluconate stock

---

6. One liter of a TPN solution is to contain 80 mEq of sodium and 30 mEq of acetate. Available stock solutions contain 4 mEq/mL sodium as sodium chloride and 2 mEq/mL sodium as sodium acetate. What quantity of each stock solution will supply the needed quantities of both ions?

- -

15 mL of sodium acetate stock; 12.5 mL of sodium chloride stock

Solution:

Acetate is the ion needed in smallest quantity (30 mEq of acetate vs. 80 mEq of sodium). Therefore, we start with sodium acetate.

$j \times 2$ mEq/mL = 30 mEq

$j = 15$ mL of sodium acetate stock solution

This also supplies 30 mEq of sodium ion. We still need 50 mEq of Na$^+$; it will come from the sodium chloride stock.

$j \times 4$ mEq/mL = 50 mEq

$j = 12.5$ mL of sodium chloride stock solution

7. A commercial electrolyte concentrate supplies the following quantities of the ions shown in terms of mEq/mL:

Sodium	0.8
Potassium	0.4
Calcium	0.096
Magnesium	0.16
Gluconate	0.096
Chloride	1.2

If 70 mL of the concentrate were used to prepare 1 L of a parenteral mixture, the amount of sodium ion would be

mEq Na^+ in concentrate = mEq Na^+ in mixture

70 mL $\times$ 0.8 mEq/mL = 56 mEq

Calculate the quantities of potassium, calcium and chloride in each liter of parenteral mixture.

_____

Potassium: 28 mEq
Calcium: 6.72 mEq
Chloride: 84 mEq

8. Most inorganic components of parenteral nutrition mixtures are specified in terms of mEq. A frequent exception is the phosphorus content, which is often described as milligrams of elemental phosphorus or millimoles of phosphate. In the body, phosphorus exists chiefly as a mixture of monobasic and dibasic forms, which differ in valence. The balance between these depends on the pH. In healthy persons, the blood pH falls within a narrow range so a calculation based on mEq is possible. However, the pH may vary from normal values in many individuals who are candidates for parenteral nutrition, making a calculation based on milliequivalents ambiguous. Using millimoles or mass units to describe phosphorus content avoids these uncertainties.
    One source of phosphorus is a potassium phosphate injection, which contains a mixture of dibasic potassium phosphate (K_2HPO_4) and monobasic potassium phosphate (KH_2PO_4). Each

milliliter of the injection contains 65.2 mg of elemental P which is equivalent to 3 mmol of P as phosphate.

What quantity of this potassium phosphate injection should be used in preparation of 5 L of a solution that is to contain 12 mmol of phosphorus in each 100 mL?

––––––––––––––––––––––––

200 mL

Solution:

P content of the injection is 3 mmol/mL

$$j \times 3 \text{ mmol/mL} = 5000 \text{ mL} \times 12 \text{ mmol/100 mL}$$

$$j = 200 \text{ mL}$$

---

9. A TPN mixture is to contain 0.22 mg of P per milliliter. How many milliliters of a sodium phosphate injection containing 93 mg of P per milliliter should be used in preparation of 3 L?

––––––––––––––––––––––––

7.1 mL

Solution:

$$j \times 93 \text{ mg/mL} = 3000 \text{ mL} \times 0.22 \text{ mg/mL}$$

$$j = 7.1 \text{ mL}$$

---

10. Dextrose is a simple sugar commonly used to supply calories for parenteral nutrition. Sterile solutions in several concentrations are available to serve as a sugar source. The calculations are similar to those we have already seen.

A TPN formula calls for dextrose, 20%. What volume of 50% dextrose injection should be utilized for each liter of the TPN formula?

_____

400 mL

Solution:

$j \times$ 50 g/100 mL = 1000 mL $\times$ 20 g/100 mL

j = 400 mL

11. A TPN formula for 2 L is to contain 25% dextrose. What volume of a 70% dextrose injection will supply the needed sugar?

_____

714 mL

Solution:

$j \times$ 70 g/100 mL = 2000 mL $\times$ 25 g/100 mL

j = 714 mL

12. Each gram of dextrose monohydrate (the usual form of this compound utilized in TPN solutions) supplies 3.4 kcal of energy. How many kilocalories would be supplied by 2 L of a 25% dextrose monohydrate solution?

———————————————————————

1700 kcal

Solution:

2000 mL × 25 g/100 mL × 3.4 kcal/g = 1700 kcal

---

13. Glycerin is sometimes used as an energy source in place of dextrose. It produces 4.32 kcal of energy per gram.

   A commercial stock solution contains various amino acids, electrolytes and 3% w/v glycerin. What is the caloric contribution of the glycerin in 100 mL of this stock solution?

———————————————————————

13 kcal

Solution:

100 mL × 3 g/100 mL × 4.32 kcal/g = 13 kcal

---

14. TPN preparations usually contain fat as an energy source. The fat is supplied in the form of an emulsion, a liquid preparation in which tiny oil globules are dispersed in a water medium. Products currently available contain either 10% fat, which supplies about 1 kcal/mL, or 20% fat, which supplies about 2 kcal/mL.

   Clinical experience with parenteral nutrition has shown that a combination of carbohydrate and fat is better tolerated and utilized than a larger quantity of either component by itself. (In addition to calories, the fat emulsion contributes essential fatty acids.)

   500 mL of a 10% fat emulsion (1.1 kcal/mL) are used to prepare 1 L of a TPN solution. Calculate the number of kilocalories contributed by the emulsion.

—————————————————————

550 kcal

Solution:

500 mL × 1.1 kcal/mL = 550 kcal

---

15. Another component of the solution described in frame 14 is 1000 mL of a solution containing 24% dextrose. What percentage of the caloric value of the two energy sources is supplied by the fat emulsion?

—————————————————————

40%

Solution:

Calories contributed by dextrose:

1000 mL × 24 g/100 mL × 3.4 kcal/g = 816 kcal

From frame 14, the fat emulsion contributes 550 kcal.

$$\frac{550}{550 + 816} = 0.40 = 40\%$$

---

16. One component of a TPN formula is a 20% fat emulsion that contributes 2 kcal/mL.

A.   What is the caloric content of 225 mL of this emulsion?
B.   How many milliliters should be used to supply 800 kcal?

—————————————————————

A. 450 kcal
B. 400 mL

---

17. The formula for a parenteral nutrition mixture calls for, among other components, 750 mL of a stock solution containing 25% dextrose. How many milliliters of a 10% fat emulsion, 1.1 kcal/mL, is needed to supply the same number of calories as the dextrose?

----

580 mL

Solution:

For the dextrose:

750 mL × 25 g/100 mL × 3.4 kcal/g = 638 kcal

For the fat emulsion:

638 kcal = 1.1 kcal/mL × j

j = 580 mL

---

18. The amount of nitrogen is frequently used as a general indication of amino acids available. 1 g of nitrogen is equivalent to between 6 and 6.5 g of amino acids (aa), depending on the preparation used. One commercial preparation that contains amino acids equivalent to 10% protein delivers 1.53 g of nitrogen/100 mL. For this product,

$$\frac{10 \text{ g aa/100 mL}}{1.53 \text{ g N/100 mL}} = \frac{6.5 \text{ g aa}}{1 \text{ g N}}$$

An amino acid formulation contains 23.8 g of nitrogen per liter. If the ratio of amino acids to nitrogen is 6.3, what is the percentage concentration of amino acids?

————————————————————

15%

Solution:

23.8 g/L = 2.38 g/100 mL

2.38 g N/100 mL × 6.3 g aa/g N = 15 g aa/100 mL

---

19. A male patient weighing 80 kg is to receive 2.5 L of a parenteral mixture every 24 hours. If his nitrogen requirement is 0.3 g/kg/day, how many milliliters of an amino acid solution containing 14 grams of nitrogen per liter should be used to prepare the mixture?

————————————————————

1710 mL

Solution:

80 kg × 0.3 g N/kg/d = 24 g N/d

24 g = j × 14 g/1000 mL

j = 1710 mL

---

20. Referring to frame 19, calculate the amount of a 10% amino acid solution that should be used to prepare the parenteral mixture. Assume that for this source, 1 g N = 6.25 g amino acids.

————————————————————

1500 mL

Solution:

$$24 \text{ g N} \times 6.25 \text{ g aa/g N} = 150 \text{ g aa}$$

$$\frac{150 \text{ g}}{10 \text{ g/100 mL}} = 1500 \text{ mL}$$

---

21. Although protein can supply calories to the body, it is most efficiently utilized for building tissue when other energy sources, namely carbohydrate and fat, are administered. This "spares" the nitrogen. The ratio of nonprotein kcal to grams of nitrogen is used as a basis for estimating protein needs in patients.

    Each liter of a stock parenteral nutrition solution supplies 260 nonprotein kcal and 16 g of amino acids. Assuming that each gram of nitrogen is equivalent to 6.25 g of amino acids, the nitrogen content is

$$\frac{16 \text{ g aa}}{6.25 \text{ g aa/g N}} = 2.56 \text{ g N}$$

and the energy:nitrogen ratio is

$$\frac{260 \text{ kcal}}{2.56 \text{ g N}} = 102 \text{ kcal/g N}$$

    What is the nonprotein kcal:nitrogen ratio for parenteral solution that contains 10% amino acids and 30% dextrose? In this solution, 1 g N = 6 g amino acids.

－－－－－－－－－－－－－－－－－－－－

61 kcal/g N

Solution:

dextrose: 30 g/100 mL $\times$ 3.4 kcal/g = 1.02 kcal/mL

N: 10 g aa/100 mL $\times \dfrac{1 \text{ g N}}{6 \text{ g aa}}$ = 0.0167 g N/mL

$$\frac{1.02 \text{ kcal/}}{0.0167 \text{ g N}} = 61 \text{ kcal/g N}$$

22. 300 mL of a 70% dextrose solution is combined with 700 mL of a solution containing 10% amino acids. The combination is to be administered at the same time as 400 mL of an emulsion containing 10% fat. For the emulsion, each milliliter delivers 1.1 kcal. For the amino acid solution, 1 g N = 6.25 g amino acids. Calculate the ratio of nonprotein calories to nitrogen overall.

_____

103 kcal/g N

Solution:

Fat: 400 mL × 1.1 kcal/mL = 440 kcal

Dextrose: 300 mL × 70 g/100 mL × 3.4 kcal/g = 714 kcal

   Total nonprotein calories = 440 kcal + 714 kcal = 1154 kcal

N: 700 mL × 10 g/100 mL × $\dfrac{1 \text{ g N}}{6.25 \text{ g aa}}$ = 11.2 g

$\dfrac{1154 \text{ kcal}}{11.2 \text{ g N}}$ = 103 kcal/g N

23. Do all of these problems before checking your answers.

A. A parenteral solution is to contain 3% amino acids. How many milliliters of a 10% amino acid stock solution should be used to prepare 4 liters of the parenteral solution?

B. A TPN solution is to contain 35 mEq of sodium ion per liter. How many milliliters of a stock solution containing 2.5 mEq of sodium (as NaCl) per mL should be used to prepare 1 L?

C. It is necessary to augment a commercial TPN solution with additional calcium ion. How many milliliters of a calcium gluconate solution, 0.45 mEq/mL should be used to supply 20 mEq of calcium ion?

D. A TPN solution is to contain the following quantities in each liter: 60 mEq of Na^+; 60 mEq of K^+; 100 mEq of acetate; 60 mEq of Cl^-; 10 of mEq Mg^{2+}. How many mL of a potassium acetate stock solution, 5 mEq/mL, will supply the potassium needed for 2 L of the TPN solution? How many mEq of acetate will the stock solution provide?

E. Referring to the previous problem, how many mL of a magnesium sulfate injection, 4 mEq/mL, will supply the magnesium needed? The formula weight of magnesium sulfate is 120.4.

F. A parenteral nutrition formula calls for 400 mg of P. What quantity of a potassium phosphate injection containing 2.1 mmol/mL phosphate should be used?

G. A TPN formula includes 22% dextrose. How many mL of a 70% dextrose injection should be used for each liter of the TPN mixture?

H. How many kilocalories will be provided by each liter of the solution made in problem G?

I. How many grams of glycerin will provide 100 kcal? Each gram of glycerin produces 4.32 kcal of energy.

J. A 20% fat emulsion yields 2.1 kcal/mL. How many mL will provide 1200 kilocalories ?

K. A total of 800 mL of the emulsion described in problem J are administered over the same time period as 2000 mL of a 20% dextrose solution. What is the ratio of calories from fat to total calories?

L. An amino acid preparation contains 40 g of amino acids per liter, equivalent to 6.5 g of nitrogen per liter. How many grams of amino acids are equivalent to each gram of nitrogen?

M. A stock preparation for parenteral nutrition contains 10 grams of amino acids per 100 mL. How many grams of nitrogen would be contained in 2.5 L if each g N = 6.25 g amino acids?

N. A patient is to receive 0.5 g/kg of nitrogen. How many mL of a 15% amino acid solution will supply the amount of nitrogen needed by a 65 kg woman if 1 g N = 6.25 g amino acids?

O. A parenteral solution contains 2% amino acids and 25% dextrose. Assuming that 1 g N = 6.25 g amino acids, calculate the ratio of nonprotein calories to nitrogen.

P. A TPN mixture consists of 750 mL of a solution containing 4.2% amino acids and 25% dextrose and 500 mL of a 10% fat emulsion. Calculate the ratio of nonprotein calories to nitrogen if each mL of the fat emulsion = 1.1 kcal and 6.25 g amino acids = 1 g N.

A. 1200 mL
B. 14 mL
C. 44.4 mL
D. 24 mL; 120 mEq of acetate

E. 5 mL
F. 6.14 mL
G. 314 mL
H. 748 kcal
I. 23.1 g
J. 571 mL
K. 55%
L. 6.15 g aa/g N
M. 40 g
N. 1350 mL
O. 265 kcal/g N
P. 236 kcal/g N

Solutions:

A. $j \times 10$ g/100 mL = 4000 mL $\times$ 3 g/100 mL

j = 1200 mL

B. $j \times 2.5$ mEq/mL = 1 L $\times$ 35 mEq/L

j = 14 mL

C. $j \times 0.45$ mEq/mL = 20 mEq

j = 44.4 mL

D. $j \times 5$ mEq/mL = 2 L $\times$ 60 mEq/L

j = 24 mL

The potassium acetate solution will contain the same number of millimoles of acetate, 120 mEq.

E. $j \times 4$ mEq/mL = 2 L $\times$ 10 mEq/L

j = 5 mL

F. 400 mg/31 mg/mmol = 12.9 mmol P

$j \times 2.1$ mmol/mL = 12.9 mmol

j = 6.14 mL

G. $j \times 70$ g/100 mL = 1000 mL $\times$ 22 g/100 mL

j = 314 mL

H. 1000 mL $\times$ 22 g/100 mL $\times$ 3.4 kcal/g = 748 kcal

I. $\dfrac{100 \text{ kcal}}{4.32 \text{ kcal/g}} = 23.1 \text{ g}$

J. $\dfrac{1200 \text{ kcal}}{2.1 \text{ kcal/mL}} = 571 \text{ mL}$

K. 800 mL × 2.1 kcal/mL = 1680 kcal from fat

2000 mL × 20 g/100 mL × 3.4 kcal/g = 1360 kcal

$\dfrac{1680}{1680 + 1360} = 0.55 = 55\%$

L. $\dfrac{40 \text{ g aa}}{6.5 \text{ g N}} = 6.15 \text{ g aa/g N}$

M. $2500 \text{ mL} \times 10 \text{ g aa/100 mL} \times \dfrac{1 \text{ g N}}{6.25 \text{ g aa}} = 40 \text{ g N}$

N. $0.5 \text{ g N/kg} \times 65 \text{ kg} \times 6.25 \text{ g aa/g N} = j \times 15 \text{ g aa/100 mL}$

$j = 1350 \text{ mL}$

O. $\dfrac{25 \text{ g/100 mL} \times 3.4 \text{ kcal/g}}{2 \text{ g aa/100 mL} \times \dfrac{1 \text{ g N}}{6.25 \text{ g aa}}} = \dfrac{0.85 \text{ kcal}}{0.0032 \text{ g N}} = 265 \text{ kcal/g N}$

P. $\dfrac{750 \text{ mL} \times 25 \text{ g/100 mL} \times 3.4 \text{ kcal/g} + 500 \text{ mL} \times 1.1 \text{ kcal/mL}}{750 \text{ mL} \times 4.2 \text{ g aa/100 mL} \times \dfrac{1 \text{ g N}}{6.25 \text{ g aa}}}$

$= \dfrac{1188 \text{ kcal}}{5.04 \text{ g N}} = 236 \text{ kcal/g N}$

CHAPTER THIRTEEN

RADIOACTIVE DECAY

Radioactive isotopes undergo changes in nuclear structure with the emission of energy. This process, called *radioactive decay*, continues until a stable isotope is formed. The rate at which nuclear change occurs is an important characteristic of a particular isotope.

Specialized units are utilized to express radioactivity and its effect on living tissues. Dosage—that is, the amount of radioactivity—is a crucial issue for radioactive substances used for diagnostic and therapeutic purposes. Because of radioactive decay, the potency of a radioactive isotope is a function of time, so that the length of time elapsed following manufacture must be taken into consideration when calculating therapeutic dosage.

Learning objectives: after completing this chapter the student should be able to

1. State the units for radioactive disintegration and convert from one set of units to another.
2. Write the equations for radioactive decay.
3. Calculate the half-life of an isotope from its decay constant (or the other way around).
4. Determine the amount of radioactive isotope remaining after an indicated period of time from a knowledge of the amount present initially and the half-life.

---

1. When identifying a particular isotope of an atom, the usual symbol is preceded by the atomic weight of the isotope. Thus

---

tritium (a radioactive isotope of hydrogen whose atomic weight is 3), would be written ^{3}H while the most common hydrogen isotope is ^{1}H. The symbol for carbon, atomic weight 14, is ^{14}C.

Write the symbol for the tin isotope with atomic weight 113.

––––––––––––––––––––––––––

^{113}Sn

---

2. When the nucleus of a radioactive atom undergoes a change, the atom is said to *decay* (to produce a different atom). Another name for this event is *radioactive disintegration*. Different atoms undergo decay by different processes, so the energy produced as a result of the process depends on the isotope involved.

    One way of describing the quantity of a particular radioactive material is through the number of disintegrations that take place in unit time, usually seconds. The reason is that the rate of decay is proportional to the amount of material present. The fundamental unit is the becquerel (Bq), which represents one disintegration per second (dps).

    1 Bq = 1 dps

    The becquerel is usually too small a unit for practical purposes, so kilo- or megabecquerels are more commonly used.

    10^3 Bq = 1 kilobecquerel (kBq)

    10^6 Bq = 1 megabecquerel (MBq) = 10^3 kBq

A. If the radioactivity of a material is 1.40×10^2 kBq, how many dps does that represent?

B. Express the radioactivity of a substance with 6.33×10^7 disintegrations per second in terms of megabecquerels.

––––––––––––––––––––––––––

A. 1.4×10^5 dps

B. 63.3 MBq

Solutions:

A. 1.40×10^2 kBq $\times$ 1000 dps/kBq = 1.4×10^5 dps

B. 6.33×10^7 dps $\times \dfrac{1 \text{ MBq}}{10^6 \text{ dps}}$ = 63.3 MBq

---

3. A second unit, older but still widely used, is the curie (Ci), defined as 3.7×10^{10} dps. As with other units, prefixes are used to scale the unit size and bring numerical values into a convenient range. For small quantities of radiation, millicuries or microcuries are commonly used.

$$1 \text{ Ci} = 1000 \text{ mCi} = 1 \times 10^6 \text{ } \mu\text{Ci} = 3.7 \times 10^{10} \text{ dps}$$

A. How many disintegrations per second are represented by a material whose activity is 9.26 mCi ?

B. If an isotope undergoes 10^7 disintegrations per minute, how many microcuries does this represent?

C. How many kBq are equivalent to 20 μCi of a radioactive substance?

- -

A. 3.43×10^8 dps

B.   4.51 μCi

C.   740 kBq

Solutions:

A. $9.26 \text{ mCi} \times \dfrac{1 \text{ Ci}}{10^3 \text{ mCi}} \times \dfrac{3.7 \times 10^{10} \text{ dps}}{1 \text{ Ci}} = 3.43 \times 10^8 \text{ dps}$

B. $\dfrac{10^7 \text{ dpm}}{1 \text{ min}} \times \dfrac{1 \text{ min}}{60 \text{ s}} = 1.67 \times 10^5 \text{ dps}$

$1.67 \times 10^5 \text{ dps} \times \dfrac{1 \text{ Ci}}{3.7 \times 10^{10} \text{ dps}} \times 10^6 \text{ } \mu\text{Ci/Ci} = 4.51 \text{ } \mu\text{Ci}$

C. $20 \text{ } \mu\text{Ci} \times \dfrac{1 \text{ Ci}}{10^6 \text{ } \mu\text{Ci}} \times 3.7 \times 10^{10} \text{ dps/Ci} \times \dfrac{1 \text{ kBq}}{1000 \text{ dps}} = 740 \text{ kBq}$

---

4.   Decay of radioisotopes occurs at a rate proportional to the number of radioactive molecules present. The following equation applies to an individual isotope:

rate of decay = λN

In this equation, N is the number of radioactive molecules at any time, t, and λ (lambda) is a rate constant that depends on the identity of the particular substance. Using the notation of differential calculus, the rate of decay can be represented as $-dN/dt$. This expression describes the change in N with time; the negative sign in front of the expression indicates that as time goes on (increases), N decreases. In the absence of the negative sign, the expression would say that the amount of radioactive substance should grow over time rather than decay.

Which of the following statements are true?

A.   The number of disintegrations per unit time is proportional to the amount of a given radioactive substance present.
B.   The number of molecules of a given isotope decreases as time goes on.

— — — — — — — — — — — — — — — — — — — —

Both statements are true.

---

5.   Calculate the λ, the decay rate constant, for an isotope if 100 kBq decays instantaneously at a rate of 0.023 MBq/year.

‒ ‒ ‒ ‒ ‒ ‒ ‒ ‒ ‒ ‒ ‒ ‒ ‒ ‒ ‒ ‒ ‒ ‒

0.23 year^{-1}

Solution:

rate of decay $= \lambda N$

$$\lambda = \frac{\text{rate of decay}}{N} = \frac{0.023 \text{ MBq/year}}{0.1 \text{ MBq}} = 0.23 \text{ year}^{-1}$$

6. In frame 5 we saw that radioactive decay could be described by this equation:

$$-\frac{dN}{dt} = \lambda N$$

This equation can be rearranged to

$$\frac{dN}{N} = -\lambda \, dt$$

and solved by integration to yield

$$N = N_0 \, e^{-\lambda t}$$

N_0 is defined as the initial number of radioactive atoms present; e is the base of natural logarithms, 2.718. Using this equation and a calculator or log table, it is possible to calculate the amount of radioactivity at any time if we know the original activity and the rate constant.

But before we do any calculations of that type, let us explore some properties of this equation by dividing both sides by N_0:

$$\frac{N}{N_0} = e^{-\lambda t}$$

The product of λ and t in this equation has to be dimensionless. Therefore the units of λ are reciprocal time (1/time). For example, if the unit of time used is seconds (s), the units of λ are expressed as 1/s usually written s^{-1}.

Write the units for λ when time is in years.

‒ ‒ ‒ ‒ ‒ ‒ ‒ ‒ ‒ ‒ ‒ ‒ ‒ ‒ ‒ ‒ ‒ ‒

$$\frac{1}{\text{year}} \text{ or year}^{-1}$$

7. We saw that the decay equation could be written

$$\frac{N}{N_0} = e^{-\lambda t}$$

Notice that the left-hand side of this equation is a ratio of numerical values. This ratio represents the fraction of radioactive atoms remaining after decay has proceeded for a given period of time, t. The right-hand sign of the equation contains a constant, λ, in addition to t. If we choose any arbitrary time period, say 1 h, the value of $e^{-\lambda t}$ will always be the same and so will N/N_0, regardless of the amount of radioactivity originally present. In other words, during any uniform time period, a constant fraction (or percentage) of the amount present at the beginning of the time period will decay.

As an illustration, let us assume that we have 100 units of a radioactive substance with a value of λ of 0.1 h^{-1}. The value of N at various times is shown in Table 13–1, along with the ratio of N values for each 10-h period of time.

Table 13–1. Calculated Values of N Over Time: $N_0 = 100$ Units; $\lambda = 0.1$ h^{-1}

Time (h)	N (arbitrary units)	Ratio*
0	100.00	
10	36.79	0.368
20	13.53	0.368
30	4.98	0.368
40	1.83	0.368

$$* \frac{\text{Number of molecules at end of 10-h period}}{\text{Number of molecules at beginning of 10-h period}}.$$

As you can see from the table, the amount of decay from 0 to 10 h is much greater than the decay from 10 to 20 h, and so on. As time goes on, the change in N becomes smaller and smaller. However, as is shown in the third column, the fraction remaining after any 10-h period is the same regardless of the value of N at the beginning of the period.

Rank the following starting quantities of ^{226}Ra in terms of the *percent* of original activity remaining after 14 weeks of storage. (Or would they all be equal?)

1) 1 kBQ

2) 2 kBQ

3) 3 kBQ

_____

Equal percentages of activity remain.

---

8. A radioactive substance loses 4.80% of its activity in 3.0 months. If the initial activity were 6.19 kBQ, predict how many kBQ will remain at the end of 6.0 months.

_____

5.61 kBQ

Solution:

After 3 months, 6.19 kBQ × 0.952 = 5.89 kBQ remain. 5.89 kBQ is the starting amount for the second 3-month period. At the end of that time, the amount remaining should be

5.89 kBQ × 0.952 = 5.61 kBQ

---

9. ^{90}Sr loses half its activity in 25 days. In how many days will the activity of 16 MBq decay to 1 MBq?

_____

100 days

Solution:

In 25 days, activity will be 8 MBq; in 50 days, 4 MBq; in 75 days, 2 MBq; in 100 days, 1 MBq.

---

10. The decay equation can be expressed in several formats. Here are three ways of writing this equation:

$$N = N_0 \, e^{-\lambda t} \tag{1}$$

$$\ln N = \ln N_0 - \lambda t \tag{2}$$

$$\log N = \log N_0 - \frac{\lambda}{2.3} t \tag{3}$$

In Eq. 2, "ln" means *natural log* (to the base e). In Eq. (3), "log" is the logarithm to base 10.

Using a calculator or log table, it is possible to predict the activity of a radioisotope after any length of time from a knowledge of the initial activity and the value of λ.

The half-life is a useful parameter that comes from these equations. The half-life is defined the length of time required for the activity to drop to one-half its initial value. At this time, $t_{0.5}$, $N = 1/2 \, N_0$. If we make these substitutions in one of the equations, the following result is obtained:

$$t_{0.5} = \frac{0.693}{\lambda}$$

From this equation we see that the half-life depends only on the value of λ. It is independent of the initial activity.

Calculate the half-life of an isotope whose λ value is 0.023 day^{-1}.

- -

30.1 days

Solution:

$$t_{0.5} = \frac{0.693}{0.023 \text{ day}^{-1}} = \textbf{30.1 days}$$

11. What is the value of the decay rate constant, λ, for an isotope whose half-life is 16 h?

- -

0.043 h^{-1}

Solution:

$$t_{0.5} = \frac{0.693}{\lambda}$$

$$\lambda = \frac{0.693}{t_{0.5}}$$

$$\lambda = \frac{0.693}{16 \text{ h}} = 0.043 \text{ h}^{-1}$$

12. If the amount of a radioactive isotope drops to half its initial value in $t_{0.5}$ h, then in another $t_{0.5}$ hours the amount will drop in half again, or in other words, to one-fourth the initial value. During the next $t_{0.5}$ hours, the amount will drop to half once more, so that one-eighth the original amount remains. It follows that the isotope will persist for an exceedingly long period of time.

The half-life of a radioisotope is 60 days. How many days will it take for 64 µCi of the isotope to drop in activity to 8 µCi?

- -

180 days

Solution:

Three half-lives are required; 3 × 60 days = 180 days.

13. Try these problems that review the concept and calculations involving half-life:

A. The decay rate constant for ^{230}Th is 9.1×10^{-6} year^{-1}. Calculate its half-life.

B. The half-life of ^{222}Rn (radon) is 3.82 days. Calculate its decay rate constant in h^{-1}.

C. The half-life of ^{210}Bi is 5 days. What percentage of a quantity of this material will remain after 10 days?

D. The half-life of ^{210}Pb is 22 years. How long would it take for 48 μCi of ^{210}Pb to decay to 1.5 μCi?

A. 7.6×10^4 years
B. 7.56×10^{-3} h
C. 25% (50% remains after 1 half-life; 25% after 2 half-lives)
D. 110 years

Solutions:

A. $t_{0.5} = \dfrac{0.693}{\lambda} = \dfrac{0.693}{9.1 \times 10^{-6} \text{ year}^{-1}} = 7.6 \times 10^4$ years

B. $\lambda = \dfrac{0.693}{3.82 \text{ days}} \times \dfrac{1 \text{ day}}{24 \text{ h}} = 7.56 \times 10^{-3} \text{ h}$

C. $0.5 \times 0.5 = 0.25 = 25\%$

D. 5 half-lives would bring the quantity down to 1/32 of the original value, from 48 μCi to 1.5 μCi.

$5 \times 22 \text{ years} = 110 \text{ years}$

---

14. When considering time periods equal in magnitude to the half-life, it is easy to calculate the amount of radioactivity remaining. For other lengths of time, the equations describing radioactive decay can be employed:

$N = N_0 \, e^{-\lambda t}$ $\qquad\qquad\qquad$ (1)

$\ln N = \ln N_0 - \lambda t$ $\qquad\qquad$ (2)

$\log N = \log N_0 - \dfrac{\lambda}{2.3} t$ $\qquad\quad$ (3)

As an example, a sample of a radioisotope whose decay rate constant is 0.02 year has an activity of 0.5 MBq. Let us calculate the activity remaining after the sample stands for 10 years.

Using Eq. (1), $N = 0.5 \text{ MBq} \times e^{-[(0.02)\,(10)]} = 0.41 \text{ MBq}$.

Using Eq. (2), $\ln N = \ln(0.5 \text{ MBq}) - (0.02 \times 10)$.

$\ln N = -0.693 - 0.2 = -0.893$

$N = 0.41 \text{ MBq}$

Using Eq. (3), $\log N = \log(0.5 \text{ MBq}) - \dfrac{0.02 \times 10}{2.3}$.

$\log N = -0.301 - 0.087 = -0.388$

$N = 0.41 \text{ MBq}$

Use any appropriate equation to predict the activity of a sample of ^{195}Au, whose half-life is 183 days, after storage for 300 days. Initially, 206 μCi are present.

66.1 µCi

Solution:

$$\lambda = \frac{0.693}{183 \text{ days}} = 0.00379 \text{ day}^{-1}$$

$$N = 206 \text{ µCi} \times e^{-[(0.00379)\ (300)]} = 66.1 \text{ µCi}$$

---

15. A radioisotope whose half-life is 82 h is stored for 6 days. If the initial activity is 72 kBq, predict the activity at the end of the storage period.

21.3 kBq

Solution:

$$\frac{0.693}{82 \text{ h}} = 0.00845 \text{ h}^{-1}$$

$$N = 72 \text{ kBq} \times e^{-[(0.00845)\ (144)]} = 21.3 \text{ kBq}$$

---

16. Do all of the following problems before checking your answers:

A. Write the symbol for cobalt isotope with an atomic weight of 57.
B. 625 µCi of an isotope are present in a container. How many MBq does this quantity represent?

C. How many millicuries are represented by 950 kBq?

D. Calculate the instantaneous rate of decay, in μCi/day, for 120 mCi of an isotope whose decay rate constant is 0.006 day^{-1}

E. What is the decay rate constant of an isotope with a half-life of 14.3 days?

F. Calculate the half-life, in seconds, of an isotope for which λ = 0.0725 h^{-1}.

G. The half-life of radioactive sodium (atomic weight 22) is 2.60 years. How long will it take for 10 mCi of this isotope to decay to 2.5 mCi?

H. Referring to the isotope in question G, how many microcuries will be left after 25 years?

I. The half-life of an isotope is 6.0 days. To what quantity will 280 kBq decay in 36 days?

J.   The half-life of an isotope is 122 days. If 1 mCi of this substance is stored for 1 year, how many μCi will remain?

- -

A. ^{57}Co
B.   23.1 MBq
C.   0.0256 mCi
D.   0.72 mCi/day
E.   0.0485 day^{-1}
F.   34,400 s
G.   5.20 years
H.   12.6 μCi
I.   4.38 kBq
J.   126 μCi

Solutions:

A.   As above.

B. $625 \, \mu Ci \times \dfrac{1 \, Ci}{10^6 \, \mu Ci} \times 3.7 \times 10^{10} \, dps/Ci = 23.1 \times 10^6 \, dps = 23.1$ MBq

C. $950 \, kBq = 950 \times 10^3 \, dps$

$950 \times 10^3 \, dps \times \dfrac{1 \, Ci}{3.7 \times 10^{10} \, dps} \times \dfrac{10^3 \, mCi}{1 \, Ci} = 0.0256 \, mCi$

D.   Rate $= \lambda N = 0.006 \, day^{-1} \times 120 \, mCi = 0.72 \, mCi/day$

E. $\lambda = \dfrac{0.693}{14.3 \, days} = 0.0485 \, day^{-1}$

F. $t_{0.5} = \dfrac{0.693}{0.0725 \, h^{-1}} = 9.56 \, h$

$9.56 \, h \times 60 \, m/h \times 60 \, s/m = 34,400 \, s$

G.   Since the final value is 1/4 the initial value, 2 half-lives must pass.

2.60 years × 2 = 5.20 years

H. $N = N_0\, e^{-\lambda t}$

$\lambda = \dfrac{0.693}{2.60 \text{ years}} = 0.267 \text{ year}^{-1}$

$N = 10 \text{ mCi} \times e^{-[(0.267)\,(25)]} = 0.0126 \text{ mCi} = 12.6 \text{ }\mu\text{Ci}$

I. 36 days represents 6 half-lives. During that time, the amount will drop to 1/64 the initial quantity.

$\dfrac{280 \text{ kBq}}{64} = 4.38 \text{ kBq}$

J. $\lambda = \dfrac{0.693}{122 \text{ days}} = 0.00568$

$N = 1000 \text{ }\mu\text{Ci} \times e^{-[(0.00568)\,(365)]} = 126 \text{ }\mu\text{Ci}$

CHAPTER FOURTEEN

RATE LAWS AND SHELF LIFE

Over the years, a number of tests have been developed to confirm the identity and purity of the many drug substances that are used to treat disease. Even if a drug is 100% pure when it is used in the preparation of a product, chemical changes typically occur over a period of time. The substances produced by these processes differ from the starting material in potency and toxicity. The rate at which drug loss occurs is of great concern; at some point in time, the residual drug concentration will drop to values below allowable limits and the product will no longer meet acceptable standards for drug content. *Shelf life* is the name given to the time period during which drug content and other characteristics remain within acceptable limits.

Learning objectives: after completing this chapter the student should be able to

1. Define what is meant by the order of a rate reaction and state the order of the two rate laws most useful in describing drug degradation.
2. Calculate the half-life of a drug given the reaction order, a rate constant, and for zero-order processes, an initial concentration.
3. Calculate the time required for 10% loss of a drug given the reaction order, a rate constant, and for zero-order processes, an initial concentration.
4. Calculate the concentration of drug remaining at a given time from a knowledge of the reaction order, initial concentration and either half-life or rate constant.

5. Given a rate constant at a specific temperature and the activation energy, calculate the rate constant at another temperature.
6. Given the shelf life based on drug content at one temperature, calculate the shelf life at another temperature.

---

1. The process of drug breakdown (also known as *drug degradation*) occurs by a variety of mechanisms that depend on the chemistry of the drug and its environment. In this and succeeding frames, we explore two simple rate laws with wide applicability.
    The names of these laws come from a fundamental rate relation, which takes the form

    $$\text{rate} \propto C^P$$

    This expression states that the rate is proportional to the drug concentration (C) raised to some power, P. The value of P identifies the *order* of the equation.
    Its origin in the case of relatively simple reactions is the number of molecules of a given reactant that participate in the reaction. In a practical sense, the assignment of order is empirical, based on the way a system behaves rather than fundamental mechanisms.
    Thus a first-order rate expression has the form

    $$\text{rate} \propto C^1 \text{ (which is the same as rate} \propto C)$$

    while a second order equation would be

    $$\text{rate} \propto C^2$$

    Write the form for a zero-order rate expression.

    _____

    $$\text{rate} \propto C^0$$

---

2. The two rate laws of interest to us are zero- and first-order. Let us rewrite the first-order expression appearing in the previous frame.

    $$\text{rate} \propto C^1$$

    To change this expression of proportionality to an equation, add a proportionality constant, k, to yield

    $$\text{rate} = k_1 C^1 = k_1 C$$

The subscript 1 is used with k to emphasize that this equation is first-order.

Write the equation (including a proportionality constant, k_0) to describe the rate of a zero-order process.

––––––––––––––––––––––––––

rate $= k_0 \, C^0 = k_0$. (Any number raised to the zero power has a value of unity.)

3. We can make these rate expressions more informative by substituting a mathematical expression for the word "rate." Using the notation of differential calculus, the rate can be represented as $-\mathrm{d}C/\mathrm{d}t$. This expression represents the change in C with time; the negative sign in front of the expression indicates that as time goes on (increases), C decreases. In the absence of the negative sign, the expression would say that drug concentration grows over time rather than dropping as degradation occurs.

Let us start with the zero-order rate equation:

$$-\frac{\mathrm{d}C}{\mathrm{d}t} = k_0$$

Integration leads to the following solution:

$$C = C_0 - k_0 \, t$$

C_0 is the initial concentration. C and C_0 are in the same units, which might, for example, be g/100 mL or mg/mL or mol/L, while t can be any valid time units (i.e., seconds, minutes, hours, days, etc.). The product of k_0 and t must have the same units as C_0, to allow one term in the equation to be subtracted from the other. k_0 therefore has the units of concentration divided by time. If C_0 is in mg/mL and t is in hours, the units of k_0 are mg/mL/h. Another way of writing this is mg mL^{-1} h^{-1}.

What units would be used for k_0 if drug concentration is expressed in moles/liter and time in days?

––––––––––––––––––––––––––

mol L^{-1} day^{-1}

4. A degradation process that follows the zero-order rate law is called a zero-order (or apparent zero-order) process. We could also say that it follows zero-order kinetics. (The word *kinetics*

refers to things in motion; in chemistry, the same word describes rates of chemical change.)

As t changes from zero (the time at which the solution is prepared), drug concentration drops from C_0; the equation allows us to calculate the value of C corresponding to any value of t. As you can see from the equation, the concentration of drug remaining in solution decreases over time in a linear fashion. This is the defining characteristic of a zero-order relationship.

If a plot of drug concentration vs. time is a straight line, what is the order of the process?

(a) zero
(b) first
(c) second

_____

Zero is correct. Linear degradation rate is synonymous with a zero-order rate law.

---

5. A drug degrades by a zero-order process with a rate constant of 0.040 mg mL^{-1} year^{-1} at 25°C. If a 0.25% w/v solution is prepared and stored at 25°C, what concentration will remain after 2 years?

_____

2.42 mg/mL (or 0.242%)

Solution:

0.25% w/v = 250 mg/100 mL = 2.5 mg/mL

$C = C_0 - k_0\, t$

$= 2.5\text{ mg/mL} - (0.040\text{ mg mL}^{-1}\text{ year}^{-1} \times 2\text{ years})$

$= 2.42\text{ mg/mL}$

6. Many degradation processes appear to follow first-order kinetics. Recall that a first-order rate law means that degradation is proportional to drug concentration.

$$-\frac{dC}{dt} = k_1 C$$

This expression should look familiar to you. It has the same form as the equation for radioactive decay. All of the mathematical properties that we studied in Chapter 13 apply here.

The three variations of the integrated equation for first-order degradation are:

$$C = C_0 e^{-k_1 t} \tag{1}$$

$$\ln C = \ln C_0 - k_1 t \tag{2}$$

$$\log C = \log C_0 - \frac{k_1}{2.3} t \tag{3}$$

Recall that "ln" refers to the natural logarithm (to the base e), while "log" refers to the logarithm to the base 10. The other symbols were defined earlier.

The units of k_1 are reciprocal time s^{-1}, h^{-1}, days^{-1}, and so on. Dividing both sides in Eq. (1) by C_0 leads to

$$\frac{C}{C_0} = e^{-k_1 t}$$

The left hand side of the equation is now a ratio of concentration values. This ratio represents the fraction of the original concentration remaining after degradation has proceeded for a given period of time, t. Over any time period chosen, the ratio C/C_0 is constant regardless of what the starting concentration, C_0, was. Over that same time period, the fraction of unchanged drug remaining will always be the same.

We have two flasks containing different concentrations of the same drug. The concentration in flask A is 0.11 molar; the concentration in flask B is 0.35 molar. If the degradation process is first-order and both flasks are stored at the same temperature for 6 months, in which will the highest percentage of initial drug remain?

Flask A
Flask B
They will be the same

—————————————————————

They will each have the same percentage of initial concentration because the degradation process is first-order.

---

7. An aqueous solution containing 1.5 mg/mL of a drug loses 6.0% of its activity in 3 months. If degradation occurs by first-order kinetics, predict how much of the drug will remain at the end of 6 months. (*Hint*: What is the concentration after 3 months? Knowing the percent retained, repeat the calculation for another 3 months.)

—————————————————————

1.33 mg/mL

Solution:

The concentration remaining at the end of 3 months is 1.5 mg/mL × 0.94 = 1.41 mg/mL. 1.41 mg/mL is the starting concentration for the second 3-month period. At the end of that time, the concentration remaining should be 1.41 mg/mL × 0.94 = 1.33 mg/mL.

---

8. The concentration of a drug in solution drops by 20% in 25 days when stored at 25°C. What concentration will remain if a 0.16 molar solution of the drug is stored under the same conditions for 75 days?

—————————————————————

0.082 molar

Solution:

The drug retains 80% of its initial concentration in each 25-day period. The concentration remaining after three such periods is 0.16 molar × 0.8 × 0.8 × 0.8 = 0.082 molar.

---

9. We have seen that the fraction of drug remaining after a given time is constant when first-order kinetics apply. One way of using this property is to ask how much time has to pass in order to bring the concentration down to a specified fraction of the original value.

   One standard way of expressing this idea is in terms of a half-life or half-time for degradation. This is the time required to bring the concentration down to 50% of its initial value. The symbol used is $t_{1/2}$, $t_{50\%}$ or $t_{0.5}$.

   The second fraction of great interest, $t_{0.9}$, relates to drug stability in manufactured products. This is the time required for the concentration to drop to 90% of its original value. For most products, 90% of original content is the point at which the end of the shelf life is reached.

   We can obtain both of these values by making the appropriate substitution in any of the rate equations. $C = 0.5\,C_0$ when $t = t_{0.5}$ and $C = 0.9\,C_0$ when $t = t_{0.9}$. When we do so, the following results are obtained:

   $$t_{0.5} = \frac{0.693}{k_1}$$

   $$t_{0.9} = \frac{0.105}{k_1}$$

   Notice that neither equation contains a concentration term; $t_{0.5}$ and $t_{0.9}$ for a first-order process are independent of the starting concentration.

   A solution containing 0.636 g/100 mL of drug is stored in a closed container at 20°C. It degrades by a first-order process and the rate constant at this temperature is 0.00215 day^{-1}. Calculate the time required for the concentration to drop to (a) 90% and (b) 50% of its initial value.

(a) 48.8 days

(b) 322 days

Solutions:

$$t_{0.9} = \frac{0.105}{k_1} = \frac{0.105}{0.00215 \text{ day}^{-1}} = 48.8 \text{ days}$$

$$t_{0.5} = \frac{0.693}{k_1} = \frac{0.693}{0.00215 \text{ day}^{-1}} = 322 \text{ days}$$

---

10. A drug in a clear solution is present at a concentration of 1.0 mg/mL after manufacture. If the half-life of the drug is 800 days, is the product's shelf life at least six months?

No. $t_{0.9}$ = 121 days.

Solution:

$$k_1 = \frac{0.693}{t_{0.5}} = \frac{0.693}{800 \text{ days}} = 0.000866 \text{ day}^{-1}$$

$$t_{0.9} = \frac{0.105}{k_1} = \frac{0.105}{0.000866 \text{ day}^{-1}} = 121 \text{ days}$$

---

11. In the previous frames we have been exploring some outstanding properties of zero- and first-order rate laws. Let us now step back and review these characteristics. Table 14–1 summarizes the important mathematical relationships.

Review the relationships in Table 14–1 and make sure that you are familiar with them. The only new items in the table are equations for $t_{0.5}$ and $t_{0.9}$ for a zero-order process. Note that both quantities are dependent on the initial concentration, in contrast to the corresponding first-order equations.

Table 14–1. Summary of Equations Describing Zero- and First-Order Rate Processes

Property	Zero-order	First-order
Rate Equation	$-\dfrac{dC}{dt} = k_0$	$-\dfrac{dC}{dt} = k_1 C$
Integrated Equation(s)	$C = C_0 - k_0 t$	$C = C_0 e^{-k_1 t}$
		$\ln C = \ln C_0 - k_1 t$
		$\log C = \log C_0 - \dfrac{k_1}{2.3} t$
$t_{0.5}$	$\dfrac{C_0}{2k_0}$	$\dfrac{0.693}{k_1}$
$t_{0.9}$	$\dfrac{C_0}{10k_0}$	$\dfrac{0.105}{k_1}$

A drug degrades in a zero-order process with a k_0 value of 1 $\mu g\ mL^{-1}\ day^{-1}$. A solution containing 2.68 mg/mL is prepared. Calculate the half-life and the time at which 90% of the initial concentration will remain.

- -

$t_{0.5}$ = 1340 days; $t_{0.9}$ = 268 days

Solution:

$$t_{0.5} = \frac{C_0}{2k_0} = \frac{2680\ \mu g/mL}{(2)\ (1\ \mu g\ mL^{-1}\ day^{-1})} = 1340\ \text{days}$$

$$t_{0.9} = \frac{C_0}{10k_0} = \frac{2680\ \mu g/mL}{(10)\ (1\ \mu g\ mL^{-1}\ day^{-1})} = 268\ \text{days}$$

12. Some numerical examples will further illustrate the patterns involved. Assume that we have a drug solution whose concentration is 1.50 mg/mL. Let us use the equations to calculate the concentrations remaining at various times for both rate processes. Table 14–2 shows values calculated from the appropriate equations while, Figure 14–1 contains plots of the same data.

Table 14–2. Concentrations Over Time for Two Drugs Whose Degradation Follows Different Kinetic Patterns

Time (days)	Concentration (mg/mL)	
	Zero-order	First-order
0	1.50	1.50
10	1.30	1.23
20	1.10	1.01
30	0.90	0.823
40	0.70	0.674
50	0.50	0.552
60	0.30	0.452
70	0.10	0.370

C_0 = 1.5 mg/mL; k_0 = 0.02 mg/mL/day; k_1 = 0.02 day^{-1}.

Note that, as expected, the zero-order plot is linear with time. At some point the concentration will drop to zero. The first-order plot is not linear. Its slope decreases over time, so that the curve drops more and more slowly toward zero as time goes on.

However, the same data for a first-order process can be replotted by taking the logarithm (base 10) of concentration and plotting it against time, as suggested by the third form of the integrated first-order equation:

$$\log C = \log C_0 - \frac{k_1}{2.3} t$$

According to this equation, when $\log C$ is plotted against t, the result will be a straight line with a slope of $k_1/2.3$ and an intercept on the vertical axis of $\log C_0$. Figure 14–2, based on the data in Table 14–2, illustrates these points.

FIGURE 14-1. KINETIC DATA FOR ZERO- AND FIRST-ORDER REACTION

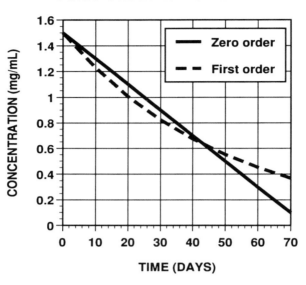

FIGURE 14-2. PLOT OF DATA FOR FIRST-ORDER KINETIC PROCESS

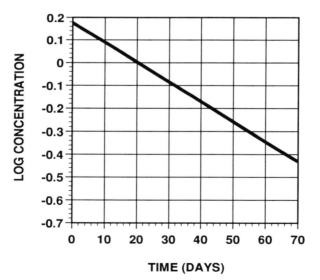

13. Chlordiazepoxide degrades in acid solution at 80°C by a first-order process. The half-life is 7 h. A 1% solution of this drug is prepared; calculate the concentration remaining (in mg/mL) after 1 h of storage at the same temperature.

_ _

9.06 mg/mL

Solution:

$$1\% = 1 \text{ g}/100 \text{ mL} = 10 \text{ mg/mL}$$

$$k_1 = \frac{0.693}{t_{0.5}} = \frac{0.693}{7 \text{ h}} = 0.099 \text{ h}^{-1}$$

$$C = C_0 \, e^{-k_1 \, t} = (10 \text{ mg/mL}) \, e^{-[(0.099) \, (1)]} = 9.06 \text{ mg/mL}$$

14. The rate constant, and therefore the reaction rate, are a function of several factors, notably pH and temperature. The *Arrhenius equation* shows the relationship between rate constant and temperature:

$$k = A \exp \left(- \frac{E_a}{R \, T} \right)$$

The notation "exp" in this equation indicates that the mathematical factor e is raised to the power that follows (in brackets). E_a is an activation energy, a parameter related to the reaction mechanism. It is assumed to be constant. R is the gas constant and T the absolute temperature. (Use of upper case distinguishes temperature from the symbol for "time.")

  If the rate constant (k) at one temperature, T, and E_a are known, the rate constant at a second temperature can be determined from the following equation form of the Arrhenius equation:

$$\log k_2 = \log k + \frac{E_a \, (T_2 - T)}{2.3 \, R \, T \, T_2}$$

where k_2 is the rate constant at the new temperature, T_2.

Let's use this equation in an example. There are a couple of things to review first. The absolute temperature, in °K, can be found by adding 273.16 to the temperature in °C. The units of E_a are typically calories/mol or joules/mol. These units may be scaled, for example to kcal/mol. The value and units of R depend on the units for E_a. If E_a is in cal/mol, R is 1.987 cal/deg/mol (cal deg^{-1} mol^{-1}); if E_a is in J/mol, R is 8.314 J/deg/mol (J deg^{-1} mol^{-1}).

The first-order degradation rate constant for a drug at 35°C is 0.092 h^{-1} (at pH 5). Calculate the rate constant at the same pH at 45°C if the activation energy is 18.0 kcal/mol.

_____

0.232 h^{-1}

Solution:

$$\log k_2 = \log k + \frac{E_a \, (T_2 - T)}{2.3 \, R \, T \, T_2}$$

$$= \log (0.092 \text{ h}^{-1})$$

$$+ \frac{(18,000 \text{ cal/mol}) \, (10 \text{ deg})}{(2.3) \, (1.987 \text{ cal deg}^{-1} \text{ mol}^{-1}) \, (308.16 \text{ deg}) \, (318.16 \text{ deg})}$$

$$\log k_2 = -1.036 + 0.402$$

$$k_2 = 0.232 \text{ h}^{-1}$$

---

15. Calculate $t_{0.5}$ at 5°C for the same compound at the same pH. (5°C approximates refrigerator temperature.)

_____

180 h

Solution:

$$\log k_2 = \log k + \frac{E_a \, (T_2 - T)}{2.3 \, R \, T \, T_2}$$

$$= \log \, (0.092) + \frac{(18,000) \, (-30)}{(2.3) \, (1.987) \, (308.16) \, (278.16)}$$

$$= -1.036 - 1.378$$

$$k_2 = 0.00385 \text{ h}^{-1}$$

$$t_{0.5} = \frac{0.693}{k_1} = \frac{0.693}{0.00385 \text{ h}^{-1}} = 180 \text{ h}$$

---

16. The rate constant for first-order degradation of a drug at 60°C is 1.67×10^{-3} h^{-1}. If the activation energy is 20.1 kcal/mol, calculate the amount remaining after storage for 200 h at 25°C. The initial concentration was 5.0 mg/mL.

- -

4.95 mg/mL

Solution:

$$\log k_2 = \log k + \frac{E_a \, (T_2 - T)}{2.3 \, R \, T \, T_2}$$

$$= \log \, (0.00167) + \frac{(20,100) \, (-35)}{(2.3) \, (1.987) \, (333.16) \, (298.16)}$$

$$= -2.777 - 1.550$$

$$k_2 = 471 \times 10^{-5} \text{ h}^{-1}$$

This is the first-order rate constant at 25°C.

$$C = C_0 \, e^{-k \, t} = (5 \text{ mg/mL}) \, e^{-[(0.0000471) \, (200)]} = 4.95 \text{ mg/mL}$$

17. The shelf life determines the expiration date that is affixed to drug products. One way to estimate shelf life is to store samples of a test batch under expected environmental conditions and determine the drug concentration periodically. When its value drops below the set specification (typically, 90% of the labeled value), the end of product life has been reached. For relatively stable formulations, this process can take several years.

We can get a good idea of the shelf life at room temperature by conducting stability tests at elevated temperatures. If exposure to higher temperatures does not introduce a new reaction, the only effect of temperature will be to increase reaction rate. Because reactions proceed much more rapidly at high temperature, the rate constant can be determined in a relatively short period of time. By determining the rate constant at several temperatures, the activation energy can be calculated. This allows extrapolation of a rate constant from an elevated temperature to the corresponding value at room temperature (or even refrigerator temperature) so that the shelf life under normal storage conditions can be projected.

As an example, the shelf life ($t_{0.9}$) for a drug at 50°C is 93 days. The activation energy for the first-order degradation process is 80,000 J/mol. To estimate the shelf life at 25°C, first calculate the rate constant at 50°C, then use the Arrhenius equation to obtain the rate constant at 25°C, and then calculate $t_{0.9}$ at that temperature.

$$k = \frac{0.105}{t_{0.9}} = \frac{0.105}{93 \text{ days}} = 0.00113 \text{ day}^{-1}$$

$$\log k_2 = \log k + \frac{E_a (T_2 - T)}{2.3 \, R \, T \, T_2}$$

$$= \log (0.00113) + \frac{(80,000) \, (-25)}{(2.3) \, (8.314) \, (323.16) \, (298.16)}$$

$$= -2.947 - 1.085 = -4.032$$

$$k_2 = 9.27 \times 10^{-5} \text{ day}^{-1}$$

$$t_{0.9} = \frac{0.105}{9.27 \times 10^{-5} \text{ day}^{-1}} = 1130 \text{ days (about 3 years)}$$

The number of steps can be reduced by substituting $0.105/t_{0.9}$ for k in the Arrhenius equation. The result is

$$\log t_{0.9(2)} = \log t_{0.9(1)} - \frac{E_a\,(T_2 - T)}{2.3\,R\,T\,T_2}$$

where $t_{0.9(2)}$ is the shelf life at the new temperature and $t_{0.9(1)}$ is the shelf life at the original temperature. You can verify that this equation is independent of the reaction order. In other words, the same equation applies to first- and zero-order reactions.

Let's try the same calculation again, using this equation:

$$\log t_{0.9(2)} = \log t_{0.9(1)} - \frac{E_a\,(T_2 - T)}{2.3\,R\,T\,T_2}$$

$$\log t_{0.9(2)} = \log (94) - \frac{(80,000)\,(-25)}{(2.3)\,(8.314)\,(323.16)\,(298.16)}$$

$$= 1.973 - (-1.085) = 3.058$$

$$t_{0.9(2)} = 1140 \text{ days}$$

Now, calculate the shelf life at 5°C.

- -

11,700 days

Solution:

$$\log t_{0.9(2)} = \log t_{0.9(1)} - \frac{E_a\,(T_2 - T)}{2.3\,R\,T\,T_2}$$

$$\log t_{0.9(2)} = \log (94) - \frac{(80,000)\,(-45)}{(2.3)\,(8.314)\,(323.16)\,(278.16)}$$

$$= 1.973 - (-2.094) = 4.067$$

$$t_{0.9(2)} = 11,700 \text{ days}$$

18. The value of $t_{0.9}$ for a drug is 35 minutes at 35°C. What is the shelf life at 5°C? The activation energy is 15.5 kcal/mol.

----

538 minutes

Solution:

$$\log t_{0.9(2)} = \log t_{0.9(1)} - \frac{E_a\,(T_2 - T)}{2.3\,R\,T\,T_2}$$

$$\log t_{0.9(2)} = \log (35) - \frac{(15{,}500)\,(-30)}{(2.3)\,(1.987)\,(308.16)\,(278.16)}$$

$$= 1.544 -(-1.187) = 2.731$$

$$t_{0.9(2)} = 538 \text{ m}$$

---

19. Here are some questions that review the material in this chapter. Try doing all of them before checking your answers.

A. The rate of a degradation of a drug is proportional to the concentration of that drug. What is the order of the reaction?

B. Write the rate equation for a degradation process that proceeds at a constant rate.

C. The rate constant for zero-order degradation of a drug is 0.860 µg mL^{-1} h^{-1} at 20°C. A 3.3% solution is prepared and stored at that temperature for 1 year. Predict the drug concentration that will be found at the end of that time.

D. What is its shelf life of the drug in question C?

E. The rate constant for digoxin degradation at 25°C at a certain
    acid pH is 2.08×10^{-4} s^{-1}. The process is first-order. Calculate the
    half-life and $t_{0.9}$ (both in minutes) of a solution at the same pH
    and temperature.

F. The half-life of a drug in aqueous solution at 25°C is 820 days. If
    degradation is a first-order process and a solution containing
    0.750 g/L is prepared, calculate the concentration remaining
    after 1 year at 25°C.

G. Referring to the drug in question F, calculate the concentration
    remaining if the same solution were stored for 1 year at 10°C.
    The activation energy for this drug is 17.4 kcal/mol.

H. A solution contains 0.25% w/v drug when freshly prepared. If the
    half-life (first-order degradation process) of the drug in this
    solution at room temperature is 12 days, predict the drug
    concentration, in mg/mL, after storage for 24 days.

I. Meperidine has a shelf life of 220 days at a pH of 3.7 and a
    temperature of 25°C. Assuming an activation energy of 19
    kcal/mol, predict the shelf life at 5°C at the same pH.

J. The degradation rate constant for a drug is 4.1×10^{-4} s^{-1} at 70°C. Assuming degradation to be apparent first-order, calculate the shelf life at this temperature.

K. Assuming the activation energy of the drug in question J is 22 kcal/mol, predict the shelf life at 25°C, in hours.

L. The half-life of a drug in solution that degrades by an apparent first-order process is 23 days. How long will it take for 10% of the drug to degrade at that temperature?

M. Referring to the drug in question L, what percentage of the initial drug present will remain after storage for 4 h?

N. The shelf life of a drug in a solution whose pH matches that of gastric fluid is 8.8 h at 5°C. An oral dose is 2 μg in 5 mL. Assuming an activation energy of 14 kcal/mol, predict the number of minutes required for unchanged drug to drop to 1.8 μg/5 mL after exposure of a dose to gastric fluid at 37°C.

————————————————————————

A. First-order
B. rate $\propto C^0$ or rate $= k_0$
C. 25,500 µg/mL = 25.5 mg/mL = 2.55%
D. 3840 h
E. $t_{0.5}$ = 55.5 min; $t_{0.9}$ = 8.4 min
F. 0.551 g/L
G. 0.703 g/L
H. 0.625 mg/mL
I. 2210 days
J. 256 s
K. 9.31 h
L. 3.49 days
M. 88.6%
N. 39 min

Solution:

A. As above.

B. As above.

C. For consistency of units, concentration is expressed in µg/mL and time in hours.

$3.3\% = 3300$ mg/100 mL = 33 mg/mL = 33,000 µg/mL

1 year = 365 days/year × 24 h/day = 8760 h

$C = C_0 - k_0 t$

$= 33,000$ µg/mL $- (0.860$ µg mL^{-1} h$^{-1} \times 8760$ h)

$= 25,500$ µg/mL

D. $t_{0.9} = \dfrac{C_0}{10 k_0} = \dfrac{33,000 \text{ µg/mL}}{(10)\,(0.860 \text{ µg mL}^{-1} \text{ h}^{-1})} = 3840$ h

E. $t_{0.5} = \dfrac{0.693}{k_1} = \dfrac{0.693}{2.08 \times 10^{-4} \text{ s}^{-1}} = 3330$ s = 55.5 min

$t_{0.9} = \dfrac{0.105}{k_1} = \dfrac{0.105}{2.08 \times 10^{-4} \text{ s}^{-1}} = 505$ s = 8.4 m

F. $k_1 = \dfrac{0.693}{t_{0.5}} = \dfrac{0.693}{820 \text{ days}} = 8.45 \times 10^{-4}$ day^{-1}

$C = C_0 e^{-k_1 t} = (0.75 \text{ g/L})\, e^{-[(0.000845)\,(365)]} = 0.551$ g/L

G. $\log k_2 = \log k + \dfrac{E_a\,(T_2 - T)}{2.3\,R\,T\,T_2}$

$= \log\,(8.45 \times 10^{-4}\ \text{day}^{-1})$

$+ \dfrac{(17{,}400\ \text{cal/mol})\,(-15\ \text{deg})}{(2.3)\,(1.987\ \text{cal deg}^{-1}\ \text{mol}^{-1})\,(298.16\ \text{deg})\,(283.16\ \text{deg})}$

$= -3.073 - 0.676$

$k_2 = 0.000178\ \text{day}^{-1}$

$C = (0.75\ \text{g/L})\ e^{-[(0.000178)\,(365)]} = 0.703\ \text{g/L}$

H. 24 days is 2 half-lives; the concentration remaining will be

2.5 mg/mL $\times$ 0.5 $\times$ 0.5 = 0.625 mg/mL

I. $\log t_{0.9(2)} = \log t_{0.9(1)} - \dfrac{E_a\,(T_2 - T)}{2.3\,R\,T\,T_2}$

$\log t_{0.9(2)} = \log\,(220) - \dfrac{(19{,}000)\,(-20)}{(2.3)\,(1.987)\,(298.16)\,(278.16)}$

$= 2.342 - (-1.003) = 3.345$

$t_{0.9(2)} = 2210\ \text{days}$

J. $t_{0.9} = \dfrac{0.105}{k_1} = \dfrac{0.105}{0.00041\ \text{s}^{-1}} = 256\ \text{s}$

K. $\log t_{0.9(2)} = \log\,(256) - \dfrac{(22{,}000)\,(-45)}{(2.3)\,(1.987)\,(343.16)\,(298.16)}$

$= 2.408 - (-2.117) = 4.525$

$t_{0.9(2)} = 33{,}500\ \text{s} = 9.31\ \text{h}$

L. $k_1 = \dfrac{0.693}{t_{0.5}} = \dfrac{0.693}{23\ \text{days}} = 0.0301\ \text{day}^{-1}$

$t_{0.9} = \dfrac{0.105}{k_1} = \dfrac{0.105}{0.0301\ \text{day}^{-1}} = 3.49\ \text{days}$

M. $C = C_0\,e^{-k_1 t} = (100\%)\,e^{-[(0.0301)\,(4)]} = 88.6\%$

N. The time required for the concentration to drop from 2 μg/5 mL to 1.8 μg/5 mL defines $t_{0.9}$.

$$\log t_{0.9(2)} = \log (8.8) - \frac{(14{,}000)\,(32)}{(2.3)\,(1.987)\,(278.16)\,(310.16)}$$

$$= 0.944 - (1.136) = -0.192$$

$$t_{0.9(2)} = 0.643 \text{ h} = 39 \text{ min}$$

APPENDIX

This appendix covers several kinds of calculations that do not fit into any of the other chapter topics or merit a chapter of their own.

I.   Temperature Conversion

Although the centigrade or Celsius scale has been used by scientists for many years and is now routinely employed in many countries as the standard means of describing temperature, the Fahrenheit scale is still in common use in the United States. Any temperature scale is arbitrary and the difference in temperature represented by "1 degree" varies from one system to another. Freezing and boiling temperatures for water are compared in Table A–1:

Table A–1. Major Points on Two Temperature Scales

Characteristic	Fahrenheit	Celsius
Boiling point of water	212°	100°
Freezing point of water	32°	0°
Difference	180°	100°

From the table we see that a difference of 180° on the Fahrenheit scale is the same as a difference of 100° on the Celsius scale. The formula for converting temperature in degrees Celsius (C) to Fahrenheit (F) is

$$°F = \frac{9}{5} °C + 32$$

By algebraic manipulation, this equation can be rearranged to

$$°C = \frac{5}{9}(°F - 32)$$

Normal body temperature is considered to be 98.6°F (although many individuals have a body temperature that is above or below this value). To convert to °C:

$$°C = \frac{5}{9}(98.6 - 32) = 37°C$$

Ordinary room temperature is about 20°C. On the Fahrenheit scale, this would be

$$°F = \frac{9}{5}(20) + 32 = 68°F$$

Try these practice problems for yourself.

A.   Convert 23°F to Celsius.

B.   Convert 177°F to Celsius.

C.   Convert –20°C to Fahrenheit.

D.   Convert 60°C to Fahrenheit.

_____

    A. $-5°C$

    B. $80.6°C$

    C. $-4°F$

    D. $140°F$

II.   Proof Strength

The standard measure of alcohol (C_2H_5OH) for purposes of taxation, is the *proof gallon*, which represents 1 gal of 50% alcohol. This strength is referred to as *proof spirit*, so that a solution containing less than 50% alcohol is "below proof," while one containing more than 50% alcohol is "above proof." The *proof strength* of alcoholic solutions is exactly double the percentage strength, v/v. Thus, proof spirit, which refers to 50% alcohol, is 100 proof, 95% alcohol is 190 proof, and 34% alcohol is 68 proof. The federal tax levied on alcohol is determined by the actual volume of C_2H_5OH contained. Thus the tax on 1 pt of 40% alcohol is equal to that on 2 pt of 20% alcohol. To compute the tax on an alcoholic solution (for payment or refund), it is necessary to dilute or concentrate the solution to 100 proof and then measure the number of gallons. Fortunately, this process takes place on paper and is not actually carried out. Our calculation involves determination of the volume of proof spirit containing the same quantity of C_2H_5OH as the solution in question.

To find the number of proof gallons, multiply the proof of the alcohol solution by the volume in gallons and divide by 100. For example, if a pharmacist has 5 gal of 30% alcohol, the number of proof gallons is

$$\frac{5 \text{ gal} \times 60}{100} = 3 \text{ proof gal}$$

The federal tax depends on the number of proof gallons. To find the federal tax (at $13.50 per proof gallon) on 2 qt of 85% alcohol, it is necessary first to determine the number of proof gallons.

$$\frac{1/2 \text{ gal} \times 170}{100} = 0.85 \text{ proof gal}$$

0.85 proof gal × \$13.50/proof gal = \$11.48

Try these problems for practice:

A.   A wine that is 29 proof contains what percentage of ethanol?

B.   How many proof gallons are equivalent to 12 gal of 25% alcohol?

C. What is the federal tax (at \$13.50 per proof gallon) on 6 gal of 70% alcohol?

D. What is the federal tax (at \$13.50 per proof gallon) on 1 pt of 72% alcohol?

E. Calculate the federal tax at 13.50 per proof gallon on 1 gal of alcohol USP, which is 95% C_2H_5OH.

_ _ _ _ _ _ _ _ _ _ _ _ _ _ _ _ _ _

A. 14.5
B. 6 proof gal
C. \$113.40
D. \$2.43
E. \$25.65

III. HLB

HLB, which stands for *hydrophile lipophile balance* is a designation applied to nonionic (uncharged) surface-active compounds. The literature accompanying commercial raw materials of this type (they are called *surfactants*) usually specifies the HLB value. It has been found over the years that certain properties of these compounds are related to their HLB value regardless of chemical makeup.

HLB is expressed as a dimensionless number. The scale ranges from zero to 20, depending on the balance between lipophilic and hydrophilic character. Real nonionic surfactants may have values from about 1 (very much toward the lipophilic side) to 19 (very much toward the hydrophilic side).

The basis of the HLB method for formulating emulsions is to match the HLB of the surfactant system with another number, called the *required HLB*, which is assigned to the oil phase of the emulsion. According to the theory, the best emulsion for a particular surfactant or mixture of surfactants is found when the surfactant HLB and the required HLB of the oil are the same. Just as the HLB numbers for surfactants are readily available, required HLB values for a number of commonly used oils have been published.

As emulsions are dispersions in which droplets of one liquid are surrounded by another, immiscible liquid, it is possible to combine these liquids so as to form two different dispersion types. One, in which oil droplets are surrounded by water, is called *oil-in-water* and abbreviated o/w. In the other type, droplets of water are surrounded by the oil. This is called *water-in-oil*, abbreviated w/o. If the surfactant HLB is below 5 or so, w/o emulsions tend to form. Higher HLB values, 10 or above, favor o/w emulsion formation.

For a mixture of surfactants, the combined HLB can be found from the individual values by the following equation:

$$HLB = \Sigma\ (f_i)\ (HLB_i)$$

f_i is the weight fraction of the ith surfactant. This is defined as the weight of that surfactant divided by the total weight of all surfactants. In a group of surfactants, the sum of all weight fractions must be 1. For two components, the equation would be

$$HLB = f_1 \times HLB_1 + f_2 \times HLB_2$$

A formula for 100 g of an emulsion contains 6 g of Span 65 (HLB = 2) and 2 g of Myrj 53 (HLB = 18). The combined HLB is

$$HLB = f_1 \times HLB_1 + f_2 \times HLB_2$$

$$\frac{6}{6+2} \times 2 + \frac{2}{6+2} \times 18 = 6$$

A similar equation applies to the required HLB of a mixture of oils:

$$RHLB = \Sigma\ (f_i)\ (RHLB_i)$$

in which RHLB is the required HLB of the mixture and $RHLB_i$ is the required HLB of the ith oil. f_i is the weight fraction of the ith oil in the oil mixture.

An emulsion contains 30 g of light mineral oil (RHLB = 12) and 6 g of another oil (RHLB = 15). The required HLB of the mixture is

$$\text{RHLB} = \Sigma \, (f_i) \, (\text{RHLB}_i)$$

$$\frac{30}{30 + 6} \times 12 + \frac{6}{30 + 6} \times 15 = 12.5$$

Two surfactants have been selected for the emulsion described above. They are polysorbate 20, with an HLB of 16.7 and sorbitan monooleate, with an HLB of 4.3. What combination of these should be used for an optimized emulsion if the total amount of surfactant to be used is 10 g? (Remember that the surfactant HLB is supposed to match the required HLB of the oil phase.)

$$\text{HLB} = f_1 \times \text{HLB}_1 + f_2 \times \text{HLB}_2$$

Let j equal the amount of polysorbate 80.

$$12.5 = \frac{j}{10} \times 16.7 + \frac{10 - j}{10} \times 4.3$$

$j = 6.6$ g of polysorbate 80

3.4 g of sorbitan monooleate would also be needed.

Try these problems for practice:

A. The HLB of sorbitan tristearate is 2.1 and that of polyoxyethylene (40) stearate is 16.9. Calculate the HLB of a 50:50 mixture of the two.

B. Referring to problem A, what is the HLB of a 5-gram mixture of the two surfactants containing 1.25 g of sorbitan tristearate?

C. The required HLB for light mineral oil in a w/o emulsion is 4; that of anhydrous lanolin is 8. What is the required HLB of the oil phase for an emulsion if it consists of 500 g of light mineral oil and 125 g of anhydrous lanolin?

D. The required HLB of the oil phase of an o/w emulsion is 13. What amounts of glyceryl monostearate (HLB = 3.8) and polysorbate 80 (HLB = 15.0) should be used if the total of the two is to be 150 g?

E. The required HLB of the oil phase of an emulsion is 10.8. What percentages of propylene glycol monostearate (HLB = 3.4) and polyethylene glycol 400 monostearate (HLB = 11.6) should be used if the total of the two surfactants is to be 8% of the total weight of the emulsion?

————————————————————————

A. 9.5
B. 13.2
C. 4.8
D. glyceryl monostearate: 26.8 g; polysorbate 80: 123.2 g
E. propylene glycol monostearate: 0.78%; polyethylene glycol 400 monostearate: 7.22%

IV. Vapor Pressure of Liquefied Propellants

Liquefied propellants are used in pressurized package systems ("aerosol" containers) to maintain constant pressure as the product is emptied. The vapor pressure is a function of temperature. In some cases, single propellants are utilized and the pressure within the product is simply the propellant's vapor pressure. When a combination of propellants is employed, each component contributes a portion of the total pressure. The partial pressure of each component may be approximated (assuming ideal behavior) as the product of the vapor pressure of the pure substance and its mole fraction. Thus

$$p_i = VP_i \times X_i$$

where p_i is the partial pressure of ingredient i, VP_i is the vapor pressure of pure i, and X_i is the mole fraction of i in the propellant mixture. The vapor pressure of the mixture is the sum of the partial pressures.

$$VP = \Sigma p_i$$

The units commonly employed in the industry are pounds per square inch gauge (psig) and pounds per square inch absolute (psia). psig is the reading that pressure gauge would indicate and represents the difference between the actual pressure and atmospheric pressure. The psia value is the actual pressure inside an aerosol container. Vapor pressures are commonly expressed in terms of psig, but all calculations should be carried out in psia. If atmospheric pressure is taken as 14.7 psi, the two units are related through the following equation:

$$psia = psig + 14.7$$

As an example, a propellant mixture is prepared by combining 150 g of propellant a, whose vapor pressure is 20 psig with 200 g of propellant b, whose vapor pressure is 45 psig. The molecular weight of propellant a is 178 while that of propellant b is 112. To calculate the mole fractions, we begin by determining the number of moles of each component:

a) $\dfrac{150\ g}{178} = 0.843$ mol

b) $\dfrac{200\ g}{112} = 1.7857$ mol

$$VP = \left((20 + 14.7) \times \frac{0.843}{0.843 + 1.7857} \right)$$

$$+ \left((45 + 14.7) \times \frac{1.7857}{0.843 + 1.7857} \right)$$

$$= 51.7\ psia = 37.0\ psig$$

Try these practice problems:

A.   What is the vapor pressure, in psig, of a mixture containing 50 g each of propellant 12 and propellant 114. Propellant 12 has a molecular weight of 121 and a vapor pressure of 84.9 psig while propellant 114 has a molecular weight of 171 and a vapor pressure of 27.6 psig.

B. What is the vapor pressure of a mixture of 20% w/w n-butane and 80% isobutane at 70°F? At this temperature, n-butane (MW 58.1) has a vapor pressure of 16.5 psig and isobutane (MW 58.1) has a vapor pressure of 30.4 psig.

C. What is the vapor pressure at 70°F of a mixture of 200 g of n-butane, 200 g of isobutane and 600 g of propane? At this temperature, propane (MW 44.1) has a vapor pressure of 110 psig. See problem B for information on the other two propellants.

_____

A. 75.9 psia = 61.2 psig
B. 42.3 psia = 27.6 psig
C. 95.6 psia = 80.9 psig

V.   Drug Binding Measured by Dialysis

Drug molecules may become attached to macromolecules, such as proteins or polymers. Dialysis is one of a series of techniques that separate molecules by size. In this technique, two chambers are separated by a semipermeable membrane. One chamber is loaded with the macromolecule, drug, water and possibly other components, such as salts. The other chamber, which we will call the receiver, contains no drug or macromolecule. Individual drug molecules of relatively low molecular weight are able to diffuse across the membrane and reach the receiver. The macromolecule, and any drug molecules bound to the macromolecule, are not.

After remaining for some time, say 24 or 48 h, the dialysis system is essentially at equilibrium. The receiver side is sampled and assayed for drug. Based on the known volume and measured concentration in the receiver, the amount of drug remaining in the first chamber can be calculated. From this, and the fact that the concentration of free (unbound) drug is the same in both chambers at equilibrium, we can determine the extent of binding. Binding is commonly expressed in two ways. One is the percentage of the drug molecules bound; the second is the amount bound per macromolecule unit.

In most dialysis apparatus, the volume of the two chambers is the same, and we will make that assumption in our calculations. As an example, the aqueous solution introduced into the left chamber of a dialysis cell contains 0.0003 mol of a polymer and 0.05 mol of a drug. The right chamber contains only water. After standing for two days, the right chamber is analyzed and found to contain 1 mmol/mL of drug. Both chambers are of equal volume, 10 mL.

Before starting the calculation, note that if no binding had occurred, the drug placed in the left chamber would have been diluted to half its concentration if all of it had been available to diffuse across the membrane. The fact that the measured concentration is less than 0.025 mol/mL tells us that some binding has taken place.

The initial amount of drug in the left chamber was 50 mmol. The amount found by assay in the right chamber (receiver) was

$$10 \text{ mL} \times 1 \text{ mmol/mL} = 10 \text{ mmol}$$

The amount remaining in the left chamber is therefore

$$50 \text{ mmol} - 10 \text{ mmol} = 40 \text{ mmol}$$

Of this quantity, 10 mmol is in equilibrium with the drug in the receiver and is therefore unbound. The amount bound is thus

$$40 \text{ mmol} - 10 \text{ mmol} = 30 \text{ mmol}$$

The percent bound is given by the amount bound divided by the total amount of drug within the left chamber

$$\frac{30 \text{ mmol}}{40 \text{ mmol}} = 75\%$$

and the binding ratio, r, defined as $\dfrac{\text{amount drug bound}}{\text{amount polymer}}$ is given by

$$r = \frac{0.03 \text{ mol drug}}{0.0003 \text{ mol polymer}} = 100 \text{ mol drug/mol polymer}$$

Here are some problems for more practice.

A.   The aqueous solution introduced into the left chamber of a
     diffusion cell contains 1.2% polyvinylpyrrolidone (PVP) and 0.30
     mmol/mL drug. The right chamber contains only water. After
     standing for 2 days, the right chamber is analyzed and found to
     contain 0.08 mmol/mL of drug. Calculate the percentage of drug
     bound in the left chamber. Both chambers are of equal volume, 12
     mL.

B.   The 50-mL chamber of a dialysis apparatus contains 0.0010 mol
     of methylcellulose (a polymer) and a drug solution, 0.10 mol/L. A
     second chamber of equal volume containing only water is
     separated from the first by a semipermeable membrane. After
     equilibration, the drug concentration in the second chamber (no
     polymer present) was found to be 0.020 molar. Calculate the
     extent of a drug binding by polymer in moles drug/mole polymer
     and the percent of drug remaining in the first chamber that is
     bound.

C.   The extent of binding of a drug to albumin, a blood protein, is
     tested by dialysis. The source solution contains a predetermined
     amount of albumin and 1 mmol/mL of a drug. After equilibration,
     the receiver is assayed and a drug concentration of 0.1 mmol/L is
     found. The volume of each chamber is 25 mL. What is the
     percentage bound?

- -

A.   64%
B.   75% bound; r = 3 mol drug/mol polymer
C.   89%

VI.   Viscosity Measurement by the Capillary Viscometer

Viscosity, the resistance of a fluid to flow, is an important parameter of many pharmaceutical products. It is one of the factors controlling the rate of sedimentation of particles in dispersions. As part of stability monitoring of drug products, viscosity can be measured over time to see whether physical changes have occurred.

The unit of viscosity in the cgs system is the poise, which is equivalent to g cm^{-1} s^{-1}. The SI unit is Pa·s (pascal seconds). For convenience, derivatives of these units are commonly used. Thus 100 cP (centipoise) = 1 poise and 1000 mPa·s (millipascal seconds) = 1 Pa·s. It is possible to convert from one set of units to the other through the following relationship:

$$1 \text{ cP} = 1 \text{ mPa·s}$$

A variety of instruments (called *viscometers*) are used to measure viscosity. For simple liquids, such as water, various oils, and glycerin, a capillary viscometer is frequently utilized. In this instrument, liquid is permitted to flow under gravity or pressure through a narrow capillary. The time required for liquid to fall between two marks is measured. For a particular volume of liquid in a particular instrument, the viscosity, η, is given by

$$\eta = K t \rho$$

where t is the measured time, ρ the liquid density and K an instrument constant that depends on a variety of factors including the geometry of the setup. The value of K can be determined by experimenting with a liquid of known density and viscosity. Once K has been determined, the same value applies for other liquids used in the same instrument under the same conditions.

The efflux time for water (ρ = 1 g/mL; η = 1 cP) in a capillary viscometer was 125 s. If the same volume of a second liquid whose density is 0.90 g/mL is placed in the same instrument and gives an efflux time of 180 s, we can calculate its viscosity by first determining K using the data for water.

$$K = \frac{\eta}{t \rho} = \frac{1}{125 \times 1} = 0.008$$

$$\eta = K t \rho = 0.008 \times 180 \times 0.90 = 1.3 \text{ cP}$$

Here are some practice problems.

A.   The efflux time for water in a capillary viscometer is 140 s. What is the viscosity of a second liquid whose efflux time in the same viscometer under the same conditions is 220 s? This liquid's specific gravity is 0.88.

B.   The time required for efflux of ethyl alcohol in a capillary viscometer is 124 s. In the same viscometer, benzyl alcohol requires 438 s. Calculate the viscosity of benzyl alcohol. The viscosity of ethanol is 1.19 cP. The specific gravity of ethanol at the temperature of measurement is 0.789. That of benzyl alcohol is 1.043.

C.   The equation for calculating viscosity from the falling ball technique is

$$\eta = K(\rho_B - \rho_L)t$$

where ρ_B is the density of the ball, ρ_L the density of the liquid and t the time required for the ball to fall a fixed distance. Using water ($\eta = 1$ cP) and a sphere of density 4.00 g/mL, the required time was 125 s. With a test liquid in the same apparatus, the same ball fell the same distance in 200 s. Calculate the viscosity of the test liquid if its density is 0.800 g/mL.

_ _

A.   1.38 cP
B.   5.56 cP = 5.56 mPa·s
C.   1.71 cP

VII.   Sedimentation Kinetics

Sedimentation rate is one aspect of the physical stability of suspensions, emulsions and other disperse systems. With certain assumptions, the rate of sedimentation, v, can be described by the *Stokes equation*:

$$v = \frac{2r^2 (\rho - \rho_0) g}{9\eta}$$

In this equation, r is the particle radius (spherical particles are assumed), ρ the density of the particle, ρ_0 the density of the medium surrounding the particle, g the acceleration of gravity (sometimes called the gravitational constant) and η the viscosity of the medium. A key assumption is that the particles not interfere with each other as they settle, so that the equation applies to dilute dispersions.

Calculate the rate of sedimentation of drug particles (26 μm diameter) in water and the time required for the suspension to settle 1 cm. (Assume that particle density is 1.5 g/mL and that the viscosity of water is 1 cP.)

Using the cgs system of units yields

$$v = \frac{2 (13 \times 10^{-4} \text{ cm})^2 (1.5 - 1 \text{ g/cm}^3) \, 980 \text{ cm}^2 \text{ s}^{-1}}{9 \times 0.01 \text{ g cm}^{-1} \text{ s}^{-1}}$$

$$= 0.018 \text{ cm/s}$$

Note that for the cgs system, viscosity is in terms of poises, with 100 cP = 1 P. Getting back to the calculation, we have

$$v = x/t$$

where x is the distance traveled and t the time.

$$t = \frac{x}{v} = \frac{1 \text{ cm}}{0.018 \text{ cm/s}} = 56 \text{ s}$$

Try these problems for practice.

A.   The density of a solid suspended in water is 1.41 g/mL. (The viscosity of water is 1.0 cP.) If the particles are of spherical shape and the same diameter, 7 μm, calculate the time required for the suspension to settle 0.5 cm.

B. Cellulose particles that are suspended in a simple water vehicle settle at a rate of 1.33 cm/h. The formulation is changed by adding sorbitol to the suspension. Calculate the length of time for the particles in the modified suspension to settle 1 cm. (The density of cellulose is 1.35 g/mL; the density and viscosity of water are 1 g/mL and 1 cP, respectively; the density and viscosity of the modified suspension medium are 1.15 g/mL and 20 cP, respectively.)

A. 457 s
B. 26 h

INDEX